HEART ATTACK

—⎍—

Will it happen to me?

HEART ATTACK

Will it happen to me?

By
Arash Bereliani, M.D., M.S., F.A.C.C.
– Associate Clinical Professor, UCLA School of Medicine
– Director, Beverly Hills Institute of Cardiology
and Preventive Medicine

CelebrityPress®
Winter Park, Florida

CONTENTS

SECTION 1
PREDICT

SECTION 2
PREVENT

SECTION 3
PIONEER

APPENDICES

ACKNOWLEDGEMENT

To my beautiful wife and my best friend, Tatiana, who has been with me through many ups and downs including the stress that accompanies writing such a book. She has been the stabilizing rock throughout my life. Her patience, understanding and acceptance of my difficult life style is incredible. She is an amazing mother to our beautiful daughter, Natasha.

To my father who inspired me to become a cardiologist and to eventually write this book and to my mother, who helped me become who I am today.

This book would not have been possible without the help of my wonderful team. A big thank you to Gabriel Green, whose genius creativity and keen ability to understand complex science and translate them into easy and understandable content, helped transfer ideas from my head and transcribe them onto paper. You truly are a genius.

Another big thank you to Sabrina Bitmayl who provided many important insights, and who helped put everything together. As usual, she was always available night and day to help with this project, and provided valuable edits and feedback.

Thanks also to Angie Swenson with the Celebrity Press who helped put my story together and was always available to guide me through this complex process. Thank you to the rest of the Celebrity Press team to help create this book including the beautiful front cover design.

Thank you to Samantha Mark who was also part of this journey and helped me see things from different perspectives.

Lastly, but not least, I would like to thank my patients throughout the last 20 years who taught me so much.

INTRODUCTION

Eight-year-old boys aren't supposed to know much about heart disease and death, but I did—not intentionally, of course. It was just another pleasant summer night, one like many in the Bereliani household that year. Summer school had just ended, and I would usually spend my summer days playing soccer with my neighbor's kids, swimming and reading books. It was a pretty regular routine. Then, every evening, we too had a routine, my brother and I. We would wait outside on the steps of our house for our dad to come home from work, while our mom cooked dinner.

Mom would insist we all have dinner together, especially on balmy summer nights such as this. And every night, like clockwork, as we waited for my dad to come home, I would always see my next-door neighbor. He would always smile at me, and very often, he would give my brother and me a candy, or sometimes a cookie. I had known him almost all my life and had developed a close bond with him and his family.

That night, however, something changed, disturbing our suburban routine. Our neighbor didn't show up. One wouldn't think that was unusual, but for him, and for us, that was something—it was everything, because he always showed up. Later on that night, we found out that he had died of a heart attack while at work. This was my first experience with the concept of death. I became depressed, refused to eat, lost weight, and couldn't fall asleep. It took me six months before I was able to get back to normal again.

Only a year later, at age nine, I nearly witnessed history repeating itself. This time, it was my own father. I watched, in abject horror, as my dad would come home and start clutching his chest in pain. As a helpless little kid, I was terrified of losing my dad the same way I had lost our next door neighbor and family friend just a year ago. My father ended up getting quintuple bypass surgery—that's five coronary arteries that were so badly blocked that they had to be "bypassed" using grafted blood vessels! And he was only in his mid-40s!

These, and many similar experiences in my childhood and teenage years, initially made me feel helpless and hopeless about this vicious killer called heart disease. It stole my next-door neighbor and very nearly took my dad. But out of the depths of helplessness developed a sense of unbridled will and fervent commitment to actually try to do something about it. That was the driving force—my motivating factor in pursuing a career in medicine. My admission essay for application to medical school was so heartfelt and genuine that I received a call from the program director to discuss it in person. She was very impressed by my desire to one day prevent heart disease.

As I continued with my training in medicine, and then with specialty training in cardiology, one question always kept nagging at me: Why—with all these advancements in the field of cardiology and medicine over the past few decades—has heart disease remained the number one cause of death, not only in the USA, but in the world? It turns out, as we shall see later, that this was not a simple question. The follow-up to this question then was: Could we live to the age of one hundred (100) without being struck down by a heart attack? These two questions have formed the basis behind my endeavors over the past 15 years.

Up until the 1970s, the only thing we, as doctors, could do for patients who had a heart attack, was to give them oxygen (which is now known not to be helpful), maybe morphine (to reduce the pain associated with the heart attack), perhaps an aspirin, and pray that they lived. If the heart attack was small, the patient might live. If, on the other hand, the heart attack was moderate or severe, the patient would have no chance of survival. That is why heart attacks were the number one killer of men and women—not only in the USA, but worldwide. We have made tremendous strides in only three to four decades since then. New advances in diagnostic testing and treatment have revolutionized the field of cardiology. Consequently, the rate of heart attacks has dropped significantly.

What is, however, still surprising (and maddeningly frustrating to cardiologists like me), is that despite all these advances in treating heart disease, in 2016, heart disease still killed more men and women, not only in the USA, but in the entire world! It killed more people than all cancers combined (including breast cancer, lung cancer, colon cancer, etc.). What is even more surprising is that most people are not aware of this fact, and seem not to worry about it as much as they do with, say, cancers. So again, we have to ask ourselves the question, why? With all these amazing technological advances in medicine, both diagnostic and therapeutic, why can we still not wipe out, or at least make heart disease the least important cause of death?

The short answer to this question is this: Everything we think we know about heart disease is partially wrong, almost everything they have told you about heart disease is wrong, and there are unspoken culprits in play that doctors don't talk about.

This book will discuss all these factors in detail and will show you why the above statements are true, but we should also address three very important factors:

First:
We developed a partial solution or treatment to the problem. Back in the 1980s, the first generation of "statin" drugs was designed to target high cholesterol levels as the primary cause of heart disease. But we now recognize that high cholesterol is only one of the contributing factors responsible for the development of heart disease.

New data that has emerged recently shows that there are a few other—and perhaps much more important factors—that we have to treat and control in order to effectively prevent heart disease. Furthermore, we now realize that many previously long-held beliefs about heart disease and cholesterol are not only incomplete but wrong. For example, not all the "bad" forms of cholesterol are bad and not all types of "good" cholesterol are good; in fact, they could be more harmful than bad cholesterol!

Second:
We, as doctors, may be to blame, although a lot of us doctors never like to admit it! What I mean is that the systematized, partitioned-off training of most doctors that doesn't emphasize prevention or multi-disciplinary collaboration, is to blame. Most cardiologists are well-versed in managing the patient who has already had a heart attack. However, most cardiologists are not well-educated and trained in how to prevent a heart attack EFFECTIVELY. Why is there this glaring disparity? Part of the reason is that—unfortunately—medical schools, residency, and fellowship institutions do not train their students on this topic.

Moreover, the field of preventive cardiology has grown just like any other modern medical specialty, but the reality is that most practitioners are not keeping up with the vast amount of knowledge that comes out almost every day in medical journals, in print and online. Between the responsibilities of bigger, corporate practices, Managed Care insurance bureaucracies, and home and family life, there just doesn't seem enough time in the day.

The "big-name, pop-culture history of cardiology" is generally written by and/or dominated by doing surgeries or procedures. Bypass surgery, heart transplants, and artificial hearts have always been, historically, what the American public knows as "practicing cardiology." Simplistic? Perhaps.

But it's reality. It is probably more exciting or satisfying to TREAT an already-developed heart attack or open a blockage of an artery than to PREVENT it. The idea of a preventive check-up is to check basic cholesterol levels, listen to their patient's heart sounds and maybe a stress treadmill test. Unfortunately, most of these tests are superficial and very useless, and they don't give the doctor any idea what their patient's risk for a heart attack is. Most cardiologists and practitioners often discuss a low fat, perhaps a low carb diet, exercise, weight loss and smoking cessation which are all relevant and useful, but barely sufficient.

Third:
The third factor causing inadequate prevention is the lack of an integrative approach to heart disease. The heart, just like other organs in our body, does not function in isolation. Every other organ and disease state can affect the heart. For example, you rarely find a patient with chronic kidney disease who has a normal, healthy heart. Our endocrine (hormone) system has a profound effect on the health of our heart. Neurological catastrophes (i.e., stroke, seizure) can cause acute or chronic heart damage. Psychiatric disturbances, rheumatological conditions, heavy metal toxicity, sleep apnea, severe anemia, etc., can have a significant and detrimental impact on the well-being of our heart.

Unfortunately, today's mainstream practitioners treat the heart as an isolated organ. How many times have you heard this from your doctor? "This is not my concern, as it relates to another part of your body, not your heart; you'll have to see another specialist for that?" There are hundreds of proven studies on how other diseases or conditions such as heavy metals, hormones, stress, rheumatological issues, kidney disease, etc. cause heart disease. The challenge here is that many of these non-cardiac conditions have no symptoms and go undiagnosed. Sometimes even mild abnormalities (which doctors don't usually treat) in these systems can affect the heart, and so are untreated.

At the start of my cardiology training, I was fortunate to get exposed to a different approach to medicine, called integrative or functional medicine. Integrative medicine is different and does not mean holistic, alternative or anti-aging medicine. It is not against using medication and doesn't use only herbal or natural supplements. This is a major misconception a great many of my patients initially had. Integrative medicine involves merely using (integrating) all the scientifically-approved modalities in the world to treat a particular disease. Traditional medicine relies very heavily on pharmaceutical medications. And think about how many "conventional medications" actually come from plants or herbs. For example: Digitalis, a significant heart medication, comes from the foxglove plant; Taxol and Taxotere, the chemotherapy drugs, from the Chinese yew tree; and even the venerable aspirin derives salicylic acid from willow bark.

Medical students are trained heavily on these medications in their pharmacology and other courses, but have no or extremely little training on any other aspects of treatment. This is, of course, due to the heavy influence of pharma in medicine. It is, for instance, not profitable (would be a loss) to run a double randomized multi-center study on vitamin C, enrolling thousands of patients to see the effect of high doses of vitamin C on various cancers, but the profits on one single new chemotherapy agent could be in the hundreds of millions or billions of dollars. Many physicians in practice are getting significantly influenced on a daily basis by different pharma reps. Mainstream (allopathic) medicine, therefore, tends to be heavily one-sided and misses many other treatments that could be very beneficial and free of side effects.

Conversely, holistic or alternative medicine tends not to be effective in treating many advanced diseases where pharmaceutical medications can be beneficial. Integrative Medicine, on the other hand, is a nice balance of the two treatment models, and if used correctly, tends to use the best of both worlds to treat disease. Integrative Medicine also uses a holistic (whole body approach) to treating a disease, which allopathic medicine fails to do.

Starting in 2004, I was exposed through some colleagues and friends to the field of integrative medicine. My initial skepticism gave way to excitement as I could see how it could be applied to the field of cardiology. In 2007, I was fully implementing what I called Integrative Cardiology in my practice. I immersed myself in learning everything there was to know to PREVENT heart disease, and introduced my integrative approach to the field of Cardiology.

The result was that over 14 years, among my large, COMPLIANT patient population with risk factors for heart disease, not even one patient developed or died of a heart attack! My method was working and proven in my own practice! I then pulled all the variables together and created a testing algorithm by which I was able to prognosticate one's risk of a heart attack with good accuracy. While my method helped, in essence, predict one's risk of a heart attack, I had to deal with another challenge: patient compliance.

We, as human beings, are a notoriously non-compliant species. How many times do doctors tell their patients to "stop smoking," "lose weight," "exercise," "eat healthy," "don't drink excessively," "take your medications regularly" and on and on and on. And how many times do we actually follow these orders for more than a few days, or at most, a few weeks? I agree part of it is that patients don't always know how, but I believe a major part has to do with complacency.

So, this was when I created the integrative treatment program. Rather than just telling the patients to "exercise" or "lose weight" or "quit smoking" or "cut down on your stress," I created an integrative treatment center right there in my offices by bringing dieticians, trainers and therapists to the patients directly. Furthermore, by embracing the latest technology, I was able to allow my patients to closely monitor their own progress with no effort. This specialized technology is now a significant part of my practice.

This book will discuss some of the real, major players (new but also some old ones) involved in a heart attack and how to prevent it with the confidence that you will live to be 100 years old without getting a heart attack. And even if you've had a heart attack before, this book will show you how to make sure you lower your risk of having another one. Remember my dad, who had the quintuple bypass in his mid-40s? Well, I'm in my mid-40s now, and my dad, I am happy and proud to say, is still very much alive.

The good news is that we now do have the most advanced technology to both diagnose heart disease at its very early stages and predict the risk of a heart attack with high accuracy. Furthermore, we have the technology to prevent and treat heart disease in its incipient stages as well. It is my firm belief that no one should develop a heart attack or die as a result of a heart attack until at least the age of 100. I believe in it because I have demonstrated this belief in my more than 15 years of practice on my own patients. So get ready to read and to live your life without a heart attack.

SECTION 1

PREDICT

CHAPTER 1

PREDICT

What if I told you that there was a method that could, in essence, predict if you were at high risk for a heart attack? Nothing special, right? You've probably heard other doctors (and other apps) talk about tests that could do the same thing. But now, what if I told you, presuming you knew that you were at high risk of having a heart attack, you could completely prevent it?

WHAT WOULD YOU DO?

Would you:

(1) **. . . want to know how to prevent it by following my recommendations, a synthesis of leading-edge predictive diagnostic techniques—founded on an evidence based, data-driven algorithm—and preventive, therapeutic interventions** that would enable you to **Head Off Heart Attacks Before They Happen?**

[Of course, that would require you to strictly follow all my medical advice including changing your lifestyle factors, such as diet and exercise, as well as taking all prescribed medications and nutritional supplements, if necessary, to prevent the impending heart attack.]

(2) **. . . rather not know when your heart attack was destined to happen?**

And just keep your head in the sand like an ostrich?

OR

(3) . . . **get angry with me either for being so bold as to** *suggest* **I could actually** *make* **such an impudent prediction,** *or* **for turning what was once merely an abstract possibility like a heart attack, into a very real** *probability*, **a concrete reality in your own personal life, complete with a timeline, in which case I sometimes become the bearer of bad news—or a combination of the two?**

You might have decided to read this book just to get some basic understanding of the heart and heart disease, or you might have picked up this book in order to figure out how to stay healthy and prevent a heart attack. Regardless of your reasons, if you are reading this book, I hope your answer is (#1), but I understand if it is (#3). Skepticism is natural, and what I am talking about is indeed bold, but it is backed up by evidence-based medicine, which is, in this case, a combination of research studies and my own experience in nearly 20 years of clinical practice. If it is (#2), I suggest you pay close attention, because ignoring the issue could have a very unfortunate outcome, not just for you, but for those you love.

Although the development of new heart medications and increased access to healthcare have produced incremental progress in the battle—from 2005 to 2015, the annual death rate attributable to coronary heart disease declined 34.4 percent and the actual number of deaths declined 17.7%. That is a deceptively rosy picture, because the burden and risk factors for cardiovascular disease remain alarmingly high. As they say these days, heart disease is still very much "a thing."

Consider these sobering statistics from the American Heart Association, published in 2018:

Cardiovascular Disease Generally (Including Heart Disease and Stroke)

- Cardiovascular disease, listed as the underlying cause of death, accounts for nearly 836,546 deaths in the USA. That's about 1 of every 3 deaths in the USA.
- About 2,300 Americans die of cardiovascular disease each day, an average of 1 death every 38 seconds.
- **Cardiovascular diseases claim more lives each year than all forms of cancer and Chronic Lower Respiratory Disease combined.**
- Coronary Heart Disease is the leading cause (43.8 percent) of deaths attributable to cardiovascular disease in the USA, followed by Stroke (16.8 percent), Heart Failure (9.0 percent), High Blood Pressure (9.4 percent), diseases of the arteries (3.1 percent), and other cardiovascular diseases (17.9 percent).

Heart Disease/Heart Attack

- **Heart Disease (including Coronary Heart Disease, Hypertension, and Stroke) remains the No. 1 cause of death in the USA.**
- **Coronary heart disease accounts for 1 in 7 deaths in the USA, killing over 366,800 people a year.**
- The overall prevalence of MI (Myocardial Infarction) in the USA is about 7.9 million, or 3 percent, in US adults.
- In 2015, heart attacks claimed 114,023 lives in the USA.
- The estimated annual incidence of heart attack in the US is 720,000 new attacks and 335,000 recurrent attacks. Average age at the first heart attack is 65.6 years for males and 72.0 years for females.
- Approximately every 40 seconds, an American will have a heart attack.

CAN WE PREDICT A HEART ATTACK?

So, can we accurately predict the chances of a heart attack?

Obviously, my answer to that question is yes—a qualified yes, but a yes nonetheless. How is this possible?

THE WHOLE BODY APPROACH

While most cardiologists look solely at cardiac-specific risk factors, a whole-body approach is required to ACCURATELY predict and treat coronary artery disease.

> *In this book, for the sake of simplicity, I shall refer to heart attack as "heart disease."*

A whole-body approach takes into account the contributions of factors such as your hormones, heavy metal toxicity, your gastrointestinal system and your emotional, mental and social health, just to name only a few. When you consider all the variables affecting your chance of getting a heart attack, you cannot ignore other parts of the body affecting your heart. Take the kidneys for example, even though your kidneys and your heart are seemingly rather far apart, as your kidney function weakens, your heart will not be far behind.

In the 1970s, the large Framingham Study shed light into some fundamental but essential risk factors contributing to heart attack: They included age, sex, high blood pressure, high cholesterol (a lot more on that later), diabetes and smoking. The Framingham Study became the model on which most predictive tools were made. Unfortunately, these risk factors even though important and valid, were only a small part of a much bigger picture which we still didn't have.

Most formulas still used today to predict one's risk of a heart attack are extremely inaccurate. Even the Framingham risk calculator which uses the data obtained from the Framingham Study to give a "10-year risk for a heart attack" is unreliable. How many friends, acquaintances or family members do you know who had a heart attack or died of sudden cardiac death without having any of the "traditional" risk factors mentioned above? How many "healthy" people do you personally know who ended up getting an angioplasty or open heart surgery?

Conversely, how many people with many of the above conditions never succumb to a heart attack or heart disease? My uncle (who was also a physician) was one of those people. While in high school, he started smoking a pack a day (the dangers of smoking had not yet been discovered in the 1940s). He continued to smoke a pack a day (sometimes more) until his early 90's and never suffered from heart disease (he passed away from pneumonia in his 90's).

What you need to understand and what this book will teach you is that our bodies are incredibly complicated. As much as we would love to try to simplify things, we have to understand that what leads to disease (in this case, a heart attack) is not as simple as adding up a few risk factors. The fat we eat doesn't just simply get stuck on the walls of our arteries and cause a heart attack! Even though the chances of getting a heart attack increase by smoking, lack of exercise and a bad diet, up until now, we could not predict when that would happen or if it would even definitively happen!

Over the past two decades, there has been an explosion in our understanding of the factors involved in causing a heart attack. We have now discovered new players which we didn't know existed when the Framingham Study was published. Furthermore, we are becoming more and more open-minded in accepting an integrative approach towards both identification and treatment of heart disease. Would you believe me if I told you that the timing of a woman's menopause can affect her risk of a heart attack? Or the many nights of binging on sushi has increased your risk of a heart attack? How about the preponderance of the harmful bacteria in your gut affecting your heart health? Or that your next door neighbor who is in perfect shape without an ounce of fat in his body and who exercises three hours a day is about to have a heart attack? These are just some examples.

The new advances in the field of preventive and integrative cardiology have enabled us to understand these newly-discovered risk factors and how to treat them. Other factors, such as loneliness and social isolation cause an increase in the stress hormone cortisol – which has been deemed to be one of the many risk factors for heart disease. How about socialization and isolation? . . . Married vs. single? Single people may not be as attentive to doctors' appointments, because quite often, a partner will drive the patient or a couple will go to the doctor together. Patients who have insomnia also have much higher rates of a heart attack as well as coronary heart disease in general.[1] If you have sleep apnea, that, unfortunately, is a very significant risk factor, and one that is very often undiagnosed, and untreated.

We all know that diabetes is a risk factor for heart disease, but what you will learn in this book is that the damage to the heart doesn't start with diabetes but in the "pre-diabetic period." As we will discuss further, pre-diabetes is practically endemic in this country. And this has contributed to a great increase in heart attack risk. Why is this? **Because we now know that the process of atherosclerosis—the formation of plaque in the arteries that leads directly and unquestionably to a heart attack—begins in the pre-diabetes stage** (a stage also referred to as **insulin resistance**).

Although most of us have a sweet tooth, we need insulin—produced by the beta cells of the pancreas—in the proper amounts to allow cells in our bodies to utilize all that glucose in our bloodstream. If there is not enough insulin, the excess sugar in our bloodstream just hangs around with nowhere to go, and you have hyperglycemia or high blood sugar. This is called **insulin resistance**. And if that state of affairs continues, it becomes diabetes.

So, glucose levels are very important. If your fasting glucose level

---

1. Javaheri S, Redline S (2017) Insomnia and Risk of Cardiovascular Disease. CHEST 152(2):435-444.

is over 90, that turns out to be a risk factor for heart attack. So are increased Hemoglobin A1C levels, which are used as a surrogate marker for diabetes or prediabetes, but which many people don't understand: They represent an average measure of your blood glucose over the life of your red blood cells, which is about three months. (Technically, the test for HbA1C measures "glycated hemoglobin," which is hemoglobin—the oxygen-carrying molecule in red blood cells—that has reacted with glucose.) But, unlike most cardiologists, I measure insulin levels too, so that I can see if there are problems with your insulin production early on, even though your glucose levels may be unaffected.

If you have a persistent HbA1C level of 6.4 or higher, you **already have** a presumptive diagnosis of coronary atherosclerosis. Of course, this is scary, but this is because we now know that the continued exposure to sustained high levels of blood glucose causes microvascular damage, that is, the interior of your arteries becomes primed and ready to form plaque deposits with lipoproteins (like LDL) in the bloodstream. The triad of high levels of blood glucose, high blood pressure, and obesity—especially central obesity, that is, visceral fat concentrated around your belly—is called the **metabolic syndrome** (it is also associated with low HDL). It is rampant throughout the United States, and it raises your risk of having a heart attack and dying from heart disease. Throw dyslipidemia (out-of-whack blood cholesterol or HDL/LDL levels) into the mix, and your risk is even higher.

HORMONES AND BIOMARKERS

Hormones

We test for **hormones**—including testosterone, estrogen, and progesterone—all of which are known to affect your heart. We, of course, test for thyroid hormones (thyroid function has a very powerful impact on the heart), insulin, and Vitamin D. (Bet you didn't know insulin and Vitamin D were hormones, did you?) Other hormones which are extremely important in heart disease include the growth hormone, cortisol, DHEA and other insulin-related hormones.

If you have read any kind of medical websites, or even medical news stories in mainstream papers and websites, in the last 20 years, you have probably heard a great deal about biomarkers, substances we can measure in the blood that can give us advanced warning of disease—in this case, heart disease. The universe of useful biomarkers has grown tremendously. Many of the biomarkers that we find interesting to measure involve those related to inflammation, for if we can identify proxies for inflammation, then we know that atherosclerotic heart disease, which sets the stage for a heart attack, cannot be too far behind. There are a number of substances which fit this description, some are well known including CRP (C-reactive protein, a general marker of inflammation) and IL-6 (interleukin-6, a proinflammatory cytokine, a type of protein that promotes inflammation in the vascular endothelium—the lining of your blood vessels where the process of atherosclerosis begins). Others are not well known, but just as important or even more important. Examples include: ST2, MCP-3 and CTACK).

GENETICS

Genetic tests are becoming increasingly important in my practice. Working with some of the top genetic-analysis laboratories in the United States, I have picked only those genetic tests that I feel have high predictive value, in both sensitivity and specificity. I have focused particularly on genes that identify people who appeared otherwise healthy (no obvious cardiac risk factors) but somehow, still had a heart attack—especially people who had episodes of unexplained sudden cardiac death (SCD). By identifying people with these genetic predispositions early, I have endeavored to try to reduce co-morbid risk factors, and thus to direct them toward the very best possible treatment.

Of course, just because you have a certain genetic profile, it is not certain you will have a heart attack. You may have a genetic predisposition to having a heart attack, but by medical interventions with diet, exercise, and medication, we can often prevent it from happening. Further, we now know that what was once thought to be set in stone (or DNA, as is the case here) genetically can now actually change. It was a given that you could not change inherited characteristics. Now we know you can. This flies in the face of 100 years of established Mendelian genetics, but it has also opened up a whole new field of study called *epigenetics.*

IMAGING

A major set of very important variables comes from what we can see through imaging technologies, which are among the state-of-the-art available, including the latest generation Cardiac CT scanners. The new advances in this technology allow not only for the detection of plaques, but it also shows the type of plaque and whether the plaque is susceptible to rupture—what we call "unstable plaque." I will discuss this in detail in the subsequent chapters in this book. Advanced carotid artery ultrasounds not only detect the earliest signs of plaque buildup, but also measure the thickness of the arterial wall, and early signs of damage to those arteries. This measure of the thickness of the arterial wall, referred to as cIMT has shown to be another important predictor of CV disease and stroke.

CAN WE LIVE TO B-100 WITHOUT SUFFERING A HEART ATTACK?

What if I told you I had a pill you could take that would let you live to 100 years of age without ever getting a heart attack, and there were no side effects. Would you take it? Obviously, you would! You'd have to be crazy not to. Well, we have that for you—only it isn't a pill. It is, however, just like a pill, based on a firm foundation of medical diagnosis and treatment—and again, supported by evidence-based medicine. Knowing what your specific genetic and biochemical risks are, and when they are likely to "trip the wires" that cause the actual heart attack will enable us to start "remodeling" you on a molecular level. This is the promise of personalized medicine. We have been hearing about it for years, but it has still not seen wide application.

The truth is, many doctors, like most of us, are creatures of habit and slow to embrace change. So are many patients. But the reality is, I have been frustrated by a medical establishment that continues to go on in a status quo mode: diagnosing and treating heart disease in essentially the same way we have for many years. We cannot continue. This means accepting patient losses due to sudden cardiac death in the hundreds of thousands per year and having heart disease remain America's leading killer—surpassing all forms of cancer, combined. It means just accepting it. Well, guess what? I don't accept it. I won't accept it and I can't accept it. And I never will.

I decided to go to medical school because I saw my next-door neighbor, who was a dear friend of the family, suddenly just not come home one night. I was told he had had a massive heart attack at work and died. I was only eight years old. Then, just a couple of years later, I witnessed my own father, clutching his chest in pain with shortness of breath. Thank God he didn't die, but he came mighty close. He had to have a quintuple bypass (that's five coronary arteries that were significantly blocked).

These things made a major impact on me as a kid. I was determined to try to stop this awful killer from taking people away in the prime of life. So, no, I do not just accept the status quo and never have. Trite as it might sound, I do want to make a difference in people's lives, and what better way to start than by making sure that more of those lives are not snuffed out prematurely by a heart attack? "What is 'prematurely,' Dr. B.?" you may ask. I contend, "Any younger than 100 years old." Overconfident? Well, I'll let you be the judge, but I ask you to read the book all the way through and consider the evidence I present before you make that judgment.

WHERE'S THE EVIDENCE THAT WE CAN LIVE TO B-100 WITHOUT HAVING A HEART ATTACK?

One piece of evidence is hidden in a small, southern Italian village nestled along the Mediterranean called Acciaroli. **Out of about 700 residents, nearly 300 of them are over 100 years of age!** Geographically speaking, these super-centenarians maintain a healthy Mediterranean diet. It goes without saying they may be working with some pretty good genes.

But researchers who have been to Acciaroli observed that these seniors also eat an amazing number of anchovies, as well as a ridiculous ration of rosemary, with their meals—much more than a standard "Mediterranean Diet." But more than that, the investigators noticed that, even though some of these people were actually overweight, and even smoked cigarettes, they were happy and remarkably stress-free. They enjoyed themselves. They looked and acted easily two decades younger. Heart disease, cancer, and diabetes were essentially non-existent.

This phenomenon is by no means limited to Acciaroli: There are places like it all over the world, everywhere from the Greek Isles to Loma Linda, California. These regions are known as "blue zones" regional communities with large populations of centenarians with "unusual" lifestyle habits.

So, based on this information, yes, I definitely believe you, too, can live to be a hundred *without having a heart attack*.

We can rebuild him. We have the technology.
~ Oscar Goldman, (1974) The Six Million Dollar Man

For my entire career as a cardiologist, I have looked for ways to better collect and analyze data, better understand the science behind heart disease, and, using whatever insights I have gained in the process, tip the odds in my patients' favor. When Oscar Goldman (played by Richard Anderson) said at the beginning of every episode of *The Six Million Dollar Man*, "We can rebuild him. We have the technology," that was science fiction. Today, it is [pretty much] scientific fact. And it won't even cost you six million dollars! (By the way, that was in 1974. Adjusted to 2018 dollars, title character Steve Austin would actually be "The 30,166,369 Dollar Man" today. Of course, there might be arguments about whether Obamacare covered his surgery. And, was Dr. Rudy Wells even in-network?)

NEW, REVOLUTIONARY FINDINGS AND THERAPIES THAT MAKE THIS ALL POSSIBLE

Advances are made by answering questions. Discoveries are made by questioning answers.
~ Bernard Haisch

Over the last 100 years, the way we treated patients with a heart attack has changed radically. For example, in the 1930s, we gave patients morphine for chest pain, maybe some digitalis, extended bed rest, and hoped for the best. We lost a lot of patients. In the 1950s, we routinely gave patients oxygen therapy and kept them in the hospital for as long as a month. We now know that this was not a good strategy, because, due to extended bed rest, blood clots would often form in the legs and the lungs, and that the oxygen therapy actually may have done more harm than good.

Today, we recognize that the first priority is to preserve heart muscle, and to identify any blood clots by performing a heart catheterization. This is usually done via an angioplasty procedure and stent placement. We can also use clot-busting drugs, such as tPA or streptokinase, to dissolve the clot. This is an example of how conventional wisdom and evidence has completely changed clinical practice.

(ALMOST) EVERYTHING YOU KNOW ABOUT PREVENTING HEART DISEASE IS WRONG!

In this book, I am going to tell you things that will probably surprise you, even shock you, because they go against everything you have heard or been taught your entire life. Most of what you have learned is wrong. And I can prove it. But I am not the only one saying them. I am just bringing them out into the open because they are not widely known. What am I talking about? Well, I'm going to explain each of these in more detail in the chapters to come, but these are some of the salient points:

- The bacteria in your gut—called the gut microbiome—determine a great deal about the health of your heart.
- Genetics has a great deal to do with your heart health, including your cholesterol level, no matter how hard you try to control it. And the amount of cholesterol you eat has fairly little to do with the amount of cholesterol that shows up in your blood.
- Heart disease has a sizable immune component. That's why we can address it with probiotics.
- Did you know that your dental health (your oral microbiome) has a profound effect on your heart health?
- Low-fat diets were a big distraction. Eating fat doesn't necessarily make you fat and doesn't cause heart attacks. The type of fat you consume is the key. Moreover, controlling your blood sugar is significantly more important.

Building on experience and observation, I adopted the position that the only way to battle heart disease successfully is to stop it before it starts. The million-dollar question became: *Could heart disease truly be prevented?* To answer that question, I had to identify and understand the root cause, and then identify a way to eliminate the threat before it reached the heart. After all, nearly every component of the human body, once compromised, will ultimately affect the heart.

I began to train closely with some of the world's foremost experts in nutraceuticals and functional medicine, while continuing to develop and build upon my passion for Cardiology through my own practice. The knowledge and experience I acquired positioned me to be one of the few cardiologists in the world to appropriately be referred to as a leading EXPERT in **preventive** and **integrative** cardiology.

> *"The most common symptom of a
> heart attack is DEATH."*

Over the last decade, there have been significant advances in preventive cardiology and the understanding of various cardiac diseases. Disturbingly, however, even with these advancements, the current methods of heart disease detection in people with no symptoms continue to fall woefully short of what is needed. As an example:

- 50% of heart attack victims have normal blood pressure levels.
- 50% of heart attack victims have normal cholesterol levels.
- 75% of stroke victims have normal blood pressure levels.

The reality of the situation is that **most cardiologists are NOT trained to prevent heart disease**. They check your cholesterol, blood pressure and a few other labs and give you medication according to the guidelines. Few cardiologists have access to the proper combination of cutting-edge technologies, or even know about it—and if they do, they probably do not know how to use it. The "stress test" utilized routinely by most physicians is a lousy and useless method to assess one's risk of a heart attack. A shocking 80% of heart-attack victims pass a stress test the day before a heart attack.

> *If these [heart health] programs really worked, heart disease
> would not remain the number 1 killer in the United States.
> Facts are facts.* ~ Dr. B

With regard to the various heart health programs that do make heart disease prevention claims, I discovered they provide the same advice, give the same medications and achieve nothing more than increased revenues.

The future of cardiovascular research is to stop the disease before it starts. It sounds simple, but we haven't really done that. What we've done before is that we identify the disease once it exists and do our best to treat it.
~ Steven Houser, Ph.D., FAHA, immediate Past President of the American Heart Association

It is my position that until cardiologists can "properly" assess all components that affect the cardiovascular system, stay up to date on all of the technical advancements and diligently monitor their patients, pharmaceutical companies will continue to be one of the top revenue-generating industries, hospital beds will remain full, and morticians will be as busy as ever.

TRANSLATING RESEARCH INTO RESULTS
The Bench-to-Bedside Continuum

After years of extensive research and refinements through clinical experience, including interactions with patients in teaching hospital settings, I have mobilized and deployed my method into my everyday private preventive and integrative cardiology practice. In so doing, I have found that no patients who diligently follow their prescribed method have died from heart disease during the entire course of therapy, and over the length of the study. I remain cautiously optimistic, but, considering that I am a cardiologist who treats some of the most complex and challenging cardiac cases. I firmly believe that heart disease is, in fact, a somewhat-predictable risk that can be avoided—or at least, managed—with proper preventive measures.

It is beyond the scope of this book to discuss every old and new risk factor in detail. Furthermore, this book is not intended to be an all-inclusive guide to diagnosing and treating heart disease. Many other conditions or treatments have not been discussed, or if so, briefly. Risk factors such as elevated Lipoprotein (a) although extremely important, has only been discussed briefly in the chapter on Genetics, and high blood pressure and smoking have not been discussed at all. Having said that, you will gain valuable insight about how heart disease develops, what affects the process and what it would take to stay free from a heart attack.

In writing this book, I had two main goals:

1. To familiarize you with some new and unheard-of risk factors and treatments in order to help you implement a healthier lifestyle, and to make you understand that you have many options when it comes to controlling the health of your heart.
2. To challenge you and change your thinking about certain incorrect beliefs, thoughts and myths that have been incorrectly installed in our minds for decades.

We will start by looking at how a heart attack occurs and the "players" involved in the process. We will discuss some common risk factors, but also some "players" you didn't know about until now (you have many surprises waiting for you). We will then talk about the role of medications, supplements and nutriceuticals. (Are they useful or a sham?) This will be followed by what kind of diet and exercise we should implement to ensure the health of our hearts (what to choose between tons of different diets and exercises out there). We will finally discuss my take on what the future of medicine holds and how medicine (in particular) will be treated in the next 5-10 years. Hope you stay with me through this exciting journey. Let's start.

CHAPTER 2

INFLAMMATION

If we are to understand a drama, we must have an accurate and up-to-date understanding of all the players involved. And obviously, I'm sure you would agree that a heart attack qualifies as a drama unlike no other. Here, we will examine the players, both old and new, and to what extent each may contribute to your heart attack risk. As we will see, whether these actors play bit or starring roles in the heart attack drama, and how much they "chew the scenery" (their relative weights in the algorithm) may determine whether your heart attack happens next week or in many years.

However, before we get to the players, we need an understanding of how a heart attack occurs. To put it simply, for the majority of heart attacks to occur, you need two things: A dysfunctional endothelium (the inner lining of the blood vessels that supply blood to the heart) which leads into plaque buildup, and in most cases, a process called Inflammation which causes the plaque to rupture. In this chapter, I will discuss these two processes in detail. Then, in the subsequent chapters of this section, we will explore the players that influence these two processes. Let's start with inflammation,

INFLAMMATION

Inflammation has also been posited as being responsible for not only cardiovascular disease, but most types of cancers, as well as neurodegenerative diseases like Alzheimer's disease. However, if inflammation were purely a bad thing, our bodies would not have evolved to develop it. You see, inflammation is actually perfectly natural.[2] A major component of the immune response, inflammation is our body's way of defending itself against damage to its cells and tissues. This damage can occur as a result of a wide variety of causes, including, but not limited to: physical injury or trauma, e.g., wounds, burns (thermal or chemical), infection (viral or bacterial), parasites, immune reactions, radiation, foreign bodies, chemical exposure, and stress.

ACUTE INFLAMMATION VS. CHRONIC INFLAMMATION

Now, I need to draw a distinction between acute inflammation and chronic inflammation. Why I do this will become clearer as we discuss the details.

Acute inflammation is signaled by a rapid onset of signs and symptoms which can commonly become severe in only a short time. However, the symptoms typically resolve in days to weeks because the inflammatory process usually eventually results in healing. Acute inflammation is often caused by an infection or an injury. Good examples include appendicitis or a wound

Chronic inflammation is typically, but not always, an unresolved acute inflammation. It may happen when your body fails to eliminate the infectious agent (usually a virus) the first time around. Its onset, in terms of any visible or perceptible signs and symptoms, is typically slow. Chronic inflammation can be

---

2. Of course, just because something is "perfectly natural" doesn't mean it's all good, either. Genetic diseases, poisons, and parasites are also "perfectly natural," too, after all!

caused by low-grade bacterial infections (which never caused symptoms previously), viral infections that were never cleared, parasites, autoimmune diseases—diseases where your body's immune system attacks normal tissue because it mistakes it for a pathogen—examples of major autoimmune diseases include Crohn's disease and rheumatoid arthritis, exposure to chemicals and environmental toxins, and radiation. Foreign bodies that have remained lodged in your body for years cause your immune system to fight back against a perceived intruder. That's chronic inflammation.

Stress is probably one of the most prevalent causes of chronic inflammation there is! Diseases that arise out of chronic inflammation include hay fever and asthma, hepatitis (transmissible), periodontal disease (the chronic inflammation here is due to poor oral hygiene), rheumatoid arthritis, ulcerative colitis/Crohn's disease—and now, what you've all been waiting for—and now, what you've all been waiting for—**atherosclerosis**, which, for those of you who did not know the definition, is the buildup of **plaque** (which is composed of fats, cholesterol, and calcium) inside the walls of your arteries. And this is why there was my huge "build up" to talking about this. Because **chronic inflammation is now the recognized mechanism for causing atherosclerosis and subsequently the rupture of the atherosclerotic plaque which in turn, is the primary driver for causing heart attacks.** We'll get back to that shortly.

What is the function of inflammation?

The *function* of inflammation, *initially*, is to:

(1) Respond to the tissue/cell damage.
(2) Remove harmful exterior stimuli.
(3) Repair the tissue damage, and, in so doing, begin the healing process.

When your little boy falls off his bicycle and skins his knee on the asphalt, or when your wife—while in the process of slicing an avocado to make that perfect guacamole for your Super Bowl party—slices her finger as well (which is actually a very common injury, by the way!). Their bodies react to these insults by an inflammatory reaction:

- First, even before inflammation, **platelets** rush to the site of the injury to stop the bleeding.[3]
- The platelets actually plug the hole in the blood vessel that is broken (and thus, bleeding) by patching the **endothelium**.

(Remember that word, boys and girls: endothelium. That's the inside cellular lining of the blood vessel, and it's really important when we're talking about heart attacks.) Now, consider that what the platelets are sensing is an interruption in the continuity of the endothelium. Just below the broken endothelium is **collagen**, one of the body's most important structural proteins, which is present in skin, bones, and connective tissue, and essential to the wound healing process—and yes, folks, this is the same collagen that is in the expensive skin creams and dermal fillers that her cosmetic dermatologist injects to diminish wrinkles. Stay with me here, this is important.

- The collagen attracts the platelets so that they can stick like glue to the vessel endothelium.
- Then, clotting factors in your blood plasma convert an inactive precursor, called fibrinogen, into its active form, **fibrin**, which creates a strong "mesh" to anchor the "platelet plug" in place. This forms the actual "blood clot."

The clot is pretty well stabilized to both the vessel wall and adjacent tissues, in this case, the skin. If it were not, and instead, broke off routinely, letting the blood clot loose into the blood

---

3. For a complete explanation of wound healing, please see Deodhar A K, Rana R E., Surgical physiology of wound healing: a review. J Postgrad Med 1997;43:52. It turns out that if you want to understand heart disease, as well as cancer, you should probably understand the process of wound healing: The growth factors that are required in the [inflammatory] processes of clotting and wound healing are the same drug targets we end up taking when it comes to trying to find innovative drug therapies for heart disease or cancer. Why? They cause inflammation and/or unwanted cell proliferation.

vessel—and therefore, into the general circulation—we would have a real problem. Now, remember I said that the platelets detect, react, and respond to, an interrupted endothelium (in our example, your kid with a skinned knee or your wife who mistakenly sliced a bit of her finger along with the avocado).[4]

I want you to consider, for a moment, what would happen if the "interrupted endothelium" wasn't *actually* "interrupted," but the platelets somehow perceived it was? A false alarm, if you will? Meaning, the blood vessel was still intact? Well, if you guessed that a clot would spontaneously form inside that blood vessel, give yourself a gold star and a pat on the back, because you'd be absolutely right.

A clot that forms inside an intact blood vessel could easily become an emergency, and sets the stage for a heart attack, stroke, or other serious cardiovascular problems. Because once that clot, or, as we cardiologists call it, a **thrombus**, finds its way to plugging another blood vessel, it then becomes a **thromboembolism**, where it can cause serious damage. A thromboembolism in the lungs is called a **pulmonary embolism**; in the blood vessels of the brain, it may lead to a **stroke**. Clots that form in, or travel to, the deep veins of the legs are a major issue, especially today, and the common term for them is **DVT** (deep venous thrombosis).

It was discovered some years ago that people who sit in an airplane seat—especially in economy class—for hours without moving are at increased risk for a DVT.[5] While DVTs used to be considered strictly the province of middle-aged and older people, younger people are increasingly becoming afflicted by them as well. The culprit? Video games on cell phones. Whereas parents used to worry that their teenagers playing their Xboxes or PlayStations for 12-hour sessions to the exclusion of family

---

4. I used the skin because it was a visually easy example for you to understand, but many damaged blood vessels are inside the body; we can't see them, and that's what makes these processes even more insidious.
5. Cruickshank JM, Gorlin R, Jennett B. Air travel and thrombotic episodes: the economy class syndrome. Lancet. 1988 Aug 27;2(8609):497-8

dinners, homework, friends, or basically anything else were simply risking poor grades and becoming socially maladjusted, now, apparently, they also need to worry about their kids developing a DVT due to sitting immobile for extended periods of time while they play their video games. This syndrome has even been given a name of its own: "gamer's thrombosis," and is being seen in patients ranging in age from teenagers to those in their 30s.[6] But I digress.

Once the bleeding is stopped, then the actual **inflammation phase** starts. Take your kid with the skinned knee on the asphalt. He probably has dirt and debris in the wound, and there are undoubtedly bacteria in there too. **Growth factors**, such as **PDGF** (platelet-derived growth factor), which are necessary to start the healing process, start to be produced. Specialized types of white blood cells called **monocytes** and **macrophages** mobilize to the area to clean up the scene, "eating up" the dead cells and debris in the wound. The macrophages actually sterilize the area by releasing reactive oxygen species, or oxygen **free radicals**[7]– which kill the bacteria.

The growth factors also do something else: they cause the growth of new blood vessels, which is known as **angiogenesis** or **neovascularization**. This is great when we are talking about healing wounds, but keep in mind for future reference that angiogenesis is not so great when we're talking about things like cancer, when the last thing you want is new blood vessels to grow so cancer cells can spread down them and establish a new beachhead, otherwise known as a metastasis. As you can see, angiogenesis is also something that must be tightly regulated, so that growth of new blood vessels is not out of control.

---

6. Chang H-CL, Burbridge H, Wong C. Extensive deep vein thrombosis following prolonged gaming ("gamer's thrombosis'): a case report. Journal of Medical Case Reports. 2013;7:235.

7. This is an example of free radicals being good, and inflammation being good, because it is solving a short-term (acute) threat to your body, which is how Nature intended the inflammation process to be used. However, a constant, years-long, assault (chronic inflammation) on your body was not what Nature intended, and the result is diseases such as cardiovascular disease and cancer.

RELATIONSHIP BETWEEN CHRONIC INFLAMMATION, PLAQUES, AND HEART ATTACKS

For years, it was thought that plaque buildup simply narrowed your arteries, blocking blood flow. It was also thought that this plaque was composed of the cholesterol that you ate, and there was simply a 1:1 correlation between your cholesterol intake and arterial plaque. In fact, coronary heart disease used to be characterized as a "cholesterol storage disease." Build up enough cholesterol-laden plaque, you block blood flow in your coronary arteries. No blood flow in your arteries equals heart attack.

Today, we know better. We now know that, after examining who actually was getting heart attacks and dying from them, *it wasn't the patients whose coronary arteries were 85-95% blocked.* Shocked? I know many of my patients were when I told them that the patients who were experiencing the *highest* morbidity and mortality from heart attacks, actually only had arteries which were less than 50% occluded by arterial plaques, but something consistent was happening: those plaques were getting ruptured. If we tested these patients on a standard stress test, it would not accurately predict the site of a future myocardial infarction (heart attack). What also was surprising was **only certain kinds of plaques were at risk for rupturing: the composition of the plaques was the determining factor**. Researchers started calling these common characteristics "vulnerable plaques."

Vulnerable plaques have:

- A soft lipid core composed of cholesterol and oxidized lipids
- A thin, fibrous cap depleted of smooth muscle cells and collagen
- Inflammatory cell infiltration — primarily by monocytes/macrophages— of the thin, fibrous cap and adventitia (the outermost connective tissue of the artery)[8]

---

8. Shah, PK, J Am Coll Cardiol, 41 (2003), pp. S15-S22.

So, we came to a rather startling conclusion: If patients had big, hard, calcified plaques, it was probably best to leave them alone. This went against all previous conventional wisdom, but the new data was starting to show us why:

The answer lay in the mechanism of inflammation.

Because **atherosclerosis is, ultimately, an immune-mediated, chronic inflammatory disease, it must be approached as one.** A kind of white blood cell, called a **monocyte**, attacks the endothelium, setting up the inflammatory response which ultimately leads to the rupture of the plaque from the endothelial surface. The plaque, which also contains **fibrin** (which is the same protein responsible for stopping bleeding) forms a clot as the plaque dislodges, causing the heart attack then and there, or an embolism downstream as it moves through the artery. The truth is, *it's an inflammation reaction that starts it all.*

So, what happens when you have chronic inflammation for years and years (and most of the time, remember, you are unaware of it, and are not being optimally treated for it). You're setting yourself up for plaque buildup in your artery walls (endothelium) and the rupture of those plaques. Scary, right? Because the body was designed to deal with short-term, acute inflammation, but not long-term (chronic) inflammation—which is what causes atherosclerosis—and a myriad of other serious health problems, including many types of cancer and, we believe, neurodegenerative diseases like Alzheimer's disease. So, reducing the burden of long-term inflammation on your body is critical.

INSIDE YOUR ARTERIES:
HOW INFLAMMATION LEADS TO A HEART ATTACK IN A FEW EASY, DEADLY, STEPS

OK, my dear devoted readers: I told you that atherosclerosis was a chronic inflammatory disease, and that your arteries didn't have to be completely blocked by plaque to have a heart attack. I also told you that certain kinds of plaques (soft, fibrous, and thin-capped) were more vulnerable to the ruptures that predisposed someone to suffer a heart attack. But what is the process by which it happens, and how is inflammation, specifically, at the root of all of it? If you don't understand that yet, don't worry. Here's where I'll take you through the steps. But before we start, let's look at the overall health of the endothelium—the lining of your blood vessels, because that's where everything begins.

ENDOTHELIAL DYSFUNCTION/ENDOTHELIAL ACTIVATION

1. **Endothelial Dysfunction.**
   Because the whole process of atherosclerosis begins in the endothelium, so do its earliest signs. So, if we see a loss of vascular tone and integrity of the endothelium, these are signs of **endothelial dysfunction**, and thus, can be an early predictor of atherosclerosis sometimes years before other clinical signs are apparent. Hypertension (high blood pressure) is also a risk factor for developing endothelial dysfunction. As a matter of fact, most of the traditional "cardiac risk factors," i.e., smoking, obesity, age, diabetes, high cholesterol, and end-stage renal disease, are all risk factors for endothelial dysfunction. So are elevated levels of the amino acid homocysteine (also a traditional heart disease risk factor). Moreover, researchers started to see characteristic changes in the dysfunctional vascular endothelium that predisposed the endothelial cells to negative outcomes such as thromboses (blood clots) down the line.

   They called processes encompassing these changes *endothelial activation*. They included (as with the definition of endothelial dysfunction) loss of vascular tone and integrity, but also added the production of leukocyte (white blood cell) adhesion molecules, a change from an antithrombotic to a prothrombotic (meaning favoring clotting of blood) phenotype, and the production of **cytokines**[9] (very important word: remember it!). Cytokines refer to a family of proteins that are perhaps best known for their role in cell signaling. Produced by the endothelium in this case, but more commonly by immune cells, such as the macrophages and monocytes we keep mentioning, often as part of an inflammatory process (although there are anti-inflammatory cytokines too), cytokines enable the next steps in the pathologic process to proceed. The net effect of endothelial activation is to loosen the barriers to the endothelium, rendering it "plump" and "leaky." Now, let's focus on a couple of critical steps. We don't know for sure in which order they may occur.

2. **Leukocyte adhesion molecules secreted by the endothelium; monocytes move on in, and morph into macrophages.**

Now that the [dysfunctional, or activated] endothelium is much more permeable, which may have happened, say, in response to various cardiac risk factors, as described above, it secretes leukocyte adhesion molecules. These allow various white blood cells, especially monocytes, to arrive on the scene. The monocytes differentiate (develop) into another kind of white cell called a **macrophage** (which literally means, in Greek, "big eater," and they definitely are!). Macrophages are extremely important in the inflammation and immunity processes, and we will be talking a great deal about them, as you will see shortly.

3. **Lipids (as lipoproteins) latch on, form lesions on subendothelium; macrophages infiltrate the area.**

The substances secreted by the endothelium have left the subendothelium (the underlayer) exposed. This is now a perfect place for lipids—especially LDL-cholesterol (the

---

9. Hunt BJ, Endothelial cell activation. A central pathophysiological process. BMJ 1998 May 2; 316(7141): 1328–1329

bad cholesterol), to latch onto. Lipids are fats. Because blood is basically water-soluble, and fats can't dissolve in water—and you need compounds to be soluble in order to do biochemical reactions—your body has to package all the fats you eat into **lipoproteins**, which, as the name might suggest, contain part lipid (fat), and part protein, so that they can then be transported throughout the bloodstream and the rest of your body. Lipoproteins contain cholesterol in addition to fat. Remember, fats are not all cholesterol. Lipoproteins can be characterized according to their density: HDL (high-density lipoprotein), LDL (low-density lipoprotein), VLDL (very low-density lipoprotein), etc.

HDL is traditionally known as "good cholesterol" (a to-help mnemonic to help you remember: H= healthy), and LDL is traditionally known as "bad cholesterol" (L=Lousy), but you must know that these are just *markers*. You must always ask your doctor whether you are measuring the number of LDL (or HDL) particles, or the amount of cholesterol associated with the particles. When we look at LDL particles (if that's the lab test your doctor ordered—which is the more expensive one), there are also characteristic patterns: It turns out that, contrary to what you might think, the *smaller, more uniform particle size* (Pattern B) *puts you at greater risk for a heart attack*! The reason for this is that these particles have an easier time penetrating the barrier of the vascular endothelium, which is protected by various defenses, including the **glycocalyx** (which we'll get to in the next chapter).

So, let's go back and look at our LDL cholesterol that has latched on to our subendothelium. Now, our LDL *particles* from our plasma can penetrate the subendothelial space, *and* remain in the *extracellular matrix* (picture them hanging out, outside the cell membrane). There, they are just ripe for oxidation.

4. **Oxidation of LDL; Incorporation of Oxidized LDL into Macrophages, Becoming Foam Cells.**
Lipids have a lot of unsaturations, or double bonds, which, when exposed to oxygen, or oxidizing conditions, will (big surprise) oxidize. These oxidized LDLs are highly reactive species, and macrophages, which are "big eaters" already, just *love* them. These "Big Macs" gobble them up, along with a bunch of cholesterol esters on the side, and they turn into something completely different: a yellowish thing called (based on its looks) a "**foam cell.**"

5. **Foam Cells Proliferate Inside the Inner layer of the Endothelium.**
Inside the inner layer of the endothelium (called the intima), proliferation of the foam cells creates a lipid-rich plaque that simply perpetuates the inflammatory process.

6. **Inflammatory Process Starts All Over Again, Creating A Destabilizing, Vulnerable Plaque.**
The whole cycle of recruitment of monocytes that differentiate into proinflammatory macrophages, which release growth factors and cytokines, starts all over again. The core of the plaque that is formed becomes necrotic (dead). Eventually, the accumulated lipoproteins in the endothelium, combined with oxidized lipids and necrotic cells, ultimately leads to the formation of soft, destabilizing, advanced lesions.

7. **Plaque progression, rupture, and heart attack.**
Progression of these plaques causes stenosis (narrowing) of affected blood vessels, which can result in angina (chest pains) and myocardial ischemia (lack of oxygen and Oxygenated blood to the heart tissues). If, however, the plaque wall is thin (referred to as a Vulnerable Plaque), it can rupture. When they do, the material inside the plaques may become exposed to prothrombotic materials in the bloodstream and a blood clot may occur, which in turn causes blocking of the blood flow to the heart and heart attack may result.

CHAPTER 3

THE GLYCOCALYX

GLYCOCALYX

I know, it sounds vaguely foreboding, like a monster from a bad science-fiction movie, but, we need to talk about it. It turns out the glycocalyx is actually one of the *good* guys in your body's defenses against heart attack. For reasons originally not well understood for many years, the endothelial glycocalyx appeared to confer a protective effect against things like "mechanical shear forces," which, it turns out, are a big factor in causing so-called endothelial dysfunction in the first place.

WHAT IS AN ENDOTHELIAL GLYCOCALYX, EXACTLY?

I know this might come as a surprise to you but one of the ways your body protects you from a heart attack or other diseases is by sugar coating you! You see **"Glycocalyx" literally means, in Greek: *"sugar coat!"***So, the endothelial glycocalyx is a sugar coat—or, more precisely, a sticky-but-slippery, gel-like barrier—composed of special sugar-based molecules—mostly glycosaminoglycans (GAGs) and proteoglycans (PGs)—which are amino sugars and sugars linked to proteins (glycoproteins)—which coats the vascular endothelium.

THERE ARE MANY ROLES PLAYED BY THE ENDOTHELIAL GLYCOCALYX

Once you see just a little bit of what we know about what its functions are, and how it works, I can practically guarantee you will agree with me that, in the words of *Family Guy*'s irrepressible Peter Griffin, this endothelial glycocalyx thing is "pretty freakin' sweet!" Let me show you why.

WHAT DOES THE ENDOTHELIAL GLYCOCALYX DO?

Think of the endothelial glycocalyx as a protective, sugary suit of clothing that every healthy, well-dressed vascular epithelium never goes out without. It functions as a powerful barrier to most things (or think of a suit that is Scotchguarded). It also acts as a signaling operations center, sending chemical messengers as needed. These messengers are called cytokines and chemokines. We'll get to those later. But, generally speaking the endothelial glycocalyx has a profound influence at the vascular wall on:

- Maintaining a selective, and thus, protective, permeability barrier between the bloodstream and the vessel wall; small molecules, lipoproteins, and blood cells are filtered out.
- Attenuating (reducing) the adhesive ability of leukocytes (white blood cells) and platelets.
- Cell-to-cell signaling and communication.
- Reducing inflammation and infection.[10]
- The transmission of shear stress (which, in turn, can cause endothelial dysfunction)

"Mechanotransduction of shear forces across the vessel wall" is something that, while perhaps not easy to conceptualize at first glance, is actually **mediated by nitric oxide (NO)**. NO mediates the transmission of shear stress across the endothelial wall (in other words, it mitigates the amount of shear stress). *And if*

---

10. Becker BF, et al., Degradation of the endothelial glycocalyx in clinical settings: searching for the sheddases. Br J Clin Pharmacol. 2015 Sep; 80(3): 389–402.

there's no NO, that could certainly upset the equilibrium of the vascular endothelium over time – enough to tip the balance in favor of what we have defined as "endothelial dysfunction."

If you remember, one thing that happens in endothelial dysfunction is the production of leukocyte adhesion molecules (see p. 45, 46 to refresh your memory). Those allow leukocytes (white blood cells) to easily adhere to the endothelial wall. This was important when we were discussing how, in the context of an injury, white blood cells (usually macrophages) could rush to the site of an injury.[11] Platelets also rush to the wound to stop the bleeding. However, these same mechanisms are also undesirable in the context of atherosclerosis.

ATHEROSCLEROSIS AND THE ENDOTHELIAL GLYCOCALYX

<u>Possibly the 1st Step in the Process!</u>
As I stated above, when the vascular endothelium itself is damaged, then, by extension, so is NO production. And that starts the whole process of an atheroma (otherwise known as an atherosclerotic lesion). In the normal state of affairs, the endothelial glycocalyx, by virtue of its slippery surface, is not hospitable to the adhesion of leukocytes, nor should there be any production of leukocyte adhesion molecules going on. In addition, there should be no pro-thrombotic compounds (substances that would cause a blood clot) being produced. Indeed, we know the endothelial glycocalyx protects against inflammation and against coagulation.

---

11. Remember, not all "inflammation" is bad: an inflammatory response is also the body's normal response to a foreign invader, which is what happens when you injure yourself, bleed, and get an infection in a wound. You want the platelets rushing to the wound site to stop the bleeding; and then, you want the white blood cells, e.g., macrophages, coming around later to debride any dead tissue, scavenge any dirt, as well as to phagocytose (a fancy word for "gobble up") any dangerous bacteria which may have colonized the wound site. However, as with many things, you just don't want too much of it, especially when that is going on in your internal organs as opposed to a little wound on your skin.

However, notwithstanding any of that, **investigators believe that your endothelial glycocalyx is your first line of defense against atherosclerosis**; or, put another way, **it's the first step on the path to an atheroma. And, it's all mediated through NO.** Because a dysfunctional endothelial glycocalyx cannot properly synthesize enough NO. Hence the path to atherosclerotic ruin.

YOUR ENDOTHELIAL GLYCOCALYX IS SHEDDING!

Further, researchers have found, through experimental evidence, that, in response to any number of "insults," i.e., damage to the endothelial glycocalyx, be they caused by inflammation [via the administration of the inflammatory cytokine TNF-alpha], trauma, surgery, sepsis, etc., or even exposure to oxidized low-density lipoprotein (LDL), the endothelial glycocalyx responds by "shedding" major known constituents of the endothelial glycocalyx from the endothelial surface. Some examples of clinical conditions which cause the glycocalyx to "shed" its constituents are: ischemia and hypoxia (very low-oxygen environments), sepsis (severe infections), inflammation, atherosclerosis, diabetes, and advanced kidney disease.[12]

A number of studies suggest that with injury or damage to the glycocalyx, certain components of the glycocalyx (such as **syndecan-1 and heparan sulfate** [13]) shed into the bloodstream. By testing for these biomarkers, we can now test for the destruction of the glycocalyx. These biomarkers may have wide application, not only for predicting cardiac problems, but even for predicting susceptibility to certain neoplastic diseases (e.g., solid tumors and certain leukemias). Some exciting evidence-based studies suggest that you may be able to reinforce, and rebuild, your endothelial glycocalyx. The way to do it could be by means of supplements to rebuild the glycosaminoglycan

---

12. Becker BF, et al., See fn. 11, supra. Br J Clin Pharmacol. 2015 Sep; 80(3): 389–402.
13. **CAUTION: Heparan sulfate ≠ Heparin!** Heparan sulfate is not the same as the heparin some people take for blood-thinning purposes.

(GAG) layer in combination with heparan sulfate, for example. Chondroitin sulfate, as you may remember, has been a popular supplement for years to rebuild cartilage in joints. Another new dietary supplement containing a seaweed extract rich in sulfated polysaccharides and glycoaminoglycans, the building blocks of the glycocalyx, have been shown to also significantly improve the damaged glycocalyx.

THE NEXT CHAPTER IS ALL ABOUT **CHOLESTEROL!**

CHAPTER 4

CHOLESTEROL

CHOLESTEROL: THE OTHER "BIG C"

I don't eat no ham 'n' eggs, 'cause they're high in cholesterol.
A yo, Phife do you eat 'em? No, Tip do you eat 'em?
Uh huh, not at all(again)
I don't eat no ham 'n' eggs, 'cause they're high in cholesterol.
Jarobi, do you eat 'em? Nope, Shah, do you eat em?
Not at all

A tisket, a tasket, what's in mama's basket?
Some veggie links and some fish that stinks.
Why, just the other day, I went to Grandma's house,
Smelled like she conjured up a mouse.
Eggs was frying, ham was smelling
In ten minutes, she started yelling (come and get it).
And the gettin's were good
I said, I shouldn't eat, she said, I think you should.
But I can't, I'm plagued by vegetarians.
No cats and dogs, I'm not a veterinarian.
Strictly collard greens and an occasional steak
Goes on my plate.
Asparagus tips look yummy, yummy, yummy
Candied yams inside my tummy

A collage of good eats, some snacks or nice treats
Apple sauce and some nice red beets.
This is what we snack on when we're Questin'
(No second guessing).

I don't eat no ham n' eggs, 'cause they're high in cholesterol
A yo, Phife do you eat 'em? No, Tip do you eat 'em?
Uh huh, not at all(again).
I don't eat no ham n' eggs, 'cause they're high in cholesterol.
Jarobi, do you eat 'em? Nope, Shah, do you eat 'em? (Nope)
Not at all.

~ A Tribe Called Quest. **"Ham 'N' Eggs"**: *People's Instinctive Travels and the Paths of Rhythm.* Jive/RCA Records, 1990.

The above lyric I quoted was from 1990, and although you may not know the song, "Ham 'N' Eggs," the group that sang it, A *Tribe Called Quest*,[14] was, according to *Rolling Stone*, one of the most influential in hip-hop and R&B music; and the album that featured "Ham 'n' Eggs" hatched hits like "I Left My Wallet In El Segundo" and "Bonita Applebum," which have been sampled by and name-checked by current superstars of the genre such as Lil Wayne and Jay-Z.

OF HIP-HOP AND HEART ATTACKS

Why, you may ask, am I quoting hip-hop lyrics in a book about heart attacks? Well, we'll get to that. I remember 1990 very well. I was an undergraduate student at UCLA, studying chemistry and biochemistry. The songs I am referring to were all over the radio. And it wasn't just African-American kids who were listening, either. It seemed like almost everybody was.

---

14. A Tribe Called Quest's 1991 follow-up album, The Low-End Theory, went platinum, yielding the smash-hit singles "Check the Rhime" and "Scenario." Their best-known founding members, Phife Dawg (real name: Malik Taylor, who referred to himself as "The Five-Footer," as he was only 5'2") and the 6'0" Q-Tip (a.k.a. Kamaal Ibn John Fareed), penned light-hearted, yet intelligent, lyrically playful rhymes about experiences that young people of all backgrounds could relate to.

I may not have been the biggest fan of rap music, but even today I recognize its place in popular culture. We remember advertising jingles and catchy lyrics like the ones to "Ham 'N' Eggs." **In this case, these lyrics reflected the conventional wisdom of the 1980s (and '70s, and '60s, and even '50s) America: that ham and eggs (especially eggs) were "high in cholesterol," and thus, were to be strenuously avoided. That cholesterol was the main root cause of heart attacks;** and that, simply by replacing foods like eggs, which were "high in cholesterol" with anything else, could reduce or eliminate one's heart attack risk. The list goes on as fad diets, wellness gurus, and even our own friends share sage, often unfounded, health advices.[15]

As a practicing cardiologist, I am sad to say that what I hear from my patients, whether in my office or in the hospital, suggests we actually don't know much better than thirty years ago when those lyrics were written.

*"Check my cholesterol, Dr. B. It should be **much** lower now that I cut out bread and rice!"*

I was surprised when I first heard that one. But no longer am I surprised how many times I hear patients who actually believe that by cutting carbs, that will affect their cholesterol level. One has absolutely nothing to do with the other. However, it is true that an excess of sugar, a carb, can cause inflammation, which is bad for blood vessels in the same way that an excess of *oxidized* LDL-cholesterol is, and the combination can have negative synergistic effects (we will discuss this in more detail in the next chapter).

The point is that most people still believe the same mistaken dietary guidelines that they heard from their parents' or grandparents' generation growing up—theories like they shouldn't eat eggs because they are "high in cholesterol." Even the weight of the evidence suggests that having some eggs now and then really should not hurt you. This is due to two main reasons:

---

15. We know oxLDL is a substrate to LDL

(1) The amount of cholesterol in a moderate number of servings of eggs does not significantly translate into an increase in total *blood* cholesterol. As I will discuss shortly, cholesterol comes from two sources: food and [mainly] what you produce internally in your liver, which is genetically determined.

(2) Total blood cholesterol is no longer even a treatment target used by the American Heart Association or the American College of Cardiology, so measuring it is of limited utility. Some of the better measures of cardiovascular disease risk where "cholesterol" is concerned are LDL-C and HDL-C scores, their subtypes, and other lipoproteins associated with them.

Phife Dawg, meanwhile, who thought he was doing the right thing by eating, and promulgating to his fans, a low-cholesterol diet, died of "complications of Type 2 diabetes" at the age of 45. He had to spend roughly the last 15 years of his life on dialysis, then a failed kidney transplant, and then dialysis again, owing to the nephropathy, or kidney damage (caused by years of damage to the blood vessels), which happens in nearly 40% of Type 2 diabetics.[16] Even though Phife Dawg was skinny when he was diagnosed (unlike the typical picture we see in Type 2 diabetes), one can deduce that **staying away from cholesterol did not help him to avoid the vascular destruction that ended his life.**

I had no access to Phife Dawg's death certificate, so I could not see his final, official cause of death, but considering that over half of all ESRD-related (end-stage renal disease) deaths are ultimately due to some form of cardiovascular disease (CVD), including heart attack, cardiac arrhythmia, or cardiac arrest, I would not be surprised if cardiovascular disease were involved. Nor would I be surprised to find extensive CVD on autopsy. This is because in the U.S., the prevalence of CVD in chronic kidney disease (CKD) patients has reached approximately 63%, compared to only 5.8% in patients without CKD (a figure nearly 9 times

---

16. Source: US National Health and Nutrition Examination Survey (NHANES) datasets, 2007-2012, overall age-adjusted CKD prevalence = 38.3%

higher than the general population).[17] In end-stage renal disease (ESRD) patients, who are, by definition, dialysis dependent (as Phife was), the risk of dying from some form of cardiovascular disease (CVD) is 10 to 20 times greater than in people without CKD.[18, 19]

We are still getting fat, having heart attacks, and experiencing diabetes even though we may be cutting out dietary cholesterol. We were told by the leading experts to eat a low-fat diet. Cut out full-fat dairy products. Saturated fats were evil. Cut out butter and choose margarine and vegetable oil and Crisco shortening instead. Remember that? Drink diet sodas and put Sweet 'N' Low in our coffee. We tried to do all that. But we still have sky-high heart-attack rates. And our society as a whole is fatter than ever.

So, what happened? What is cholesterol, really, anyway?

We talk about it all the time. We vilify it constantly, but most people know little to nothing about it.

Cholesterol is the most highly decorated small molecule in biology. Thirteen Nobel Prizes have been awarded to scientists who devoted major parts of their careers to cholesterol. Ever since it was isolated from gallstones in 1784, cholesterol has exerted an almost hypnotic fascination for scientists from the most diverse areas of science and medicine.... Cholesterol is a Janus-faced molecule.[20] **The very property that makes it useful in cell membranes, namely its absolute insolubility in water, also makes it lethal.**
~ Michael Brown and Joseph Goldstein
Nobel Lectures (1985) © The Nobel Foundation, 1985

17. Gaita D, Mihaescu A, Schiller A. Of heart and kidney:a complicated love story. Eur J Prev Cardiol.2012; 21: 840-846.

18. Foley Rn, Parfrey Ps, Sarnak MJ. Clinical epidemiology of cardiovascular disease in chronic renal disease. Am J Kidney Dis 1998; 32: S112-119.

19. Johnson Dw, Craven Am, Isbel Nm. Modification of cardiovascular risk in hemodialysis patients: An evidence-based review. Hemodial Int 2007; 11: 1-14.

20. Janus-faced molecule: a molecule which is "two-faced," i.e., has two totally opposite and contradictory effects, one usually salutary, the other deleterious (as in the Roman god of doors, Janus, usually depicted with two opposing faces).

From the word *cholesterol* itself, the Greek prefix *chole-* (as in *cholecystectomy, cholangiogram, cholecystokinin*, and even the deadly disease, *cholera*) tells us it has something to do with bile or the gallbladder. (If you're about to object to one of those words on the list, I know: Although "cholera" has nothing to do with bile, the old-time doctors used to *think* it did.) Indeed, as Nobelists Michael Brown and Joseph Goldstein told us in the above-italicized quote, cholesterol was first discovered in gallstones, which are made of bile, and, of course, form in the gallbladder. The other part of the word cholesterol is sterol, meaning a steroid alcohol.

Etymologically, the word sterol actually came from cholesterol. The word steroid, in this context, does not mean what you might think (the "anabolic steroids," which are, in fact, synthetic testosterone derivatives). They are used by weightlifters to bulk up their muscles artificially. However, as we will see, they are actually not that different from a structural point of view! By "steroid," I mean "any of a large class of organic compounds with a characteristic molecular structure containing four rings of carbon atoms (three six-membered and one five). They include many hormones, alkaloids, and vitamins." (Oxford English Dictionary.) [*See Appendix A (p. 193) for an in-depth discussion of cholesterol.*]

Cholesterol comes from two sources: (1) What you eat, and (2) What your liver synthesizes (determined genetically).

In our bodies, a couple of steps of enzymatic magic turn cholesterol into the sex hormones testosterone, DHEA, progesterone, estradiol, and aldosterone (a *mineralocorticoid*, critical for renal health and blood pressure). Other enzymes convert cholesterol into *glucocorticoids*, such as the stress hormone cortisol, made in the adrenal glands, which can be made into cortisone and hydrocortisone.

Now, remember the quote about cholesterol and its insolubility making it lethal? That's because it's just accumulating in the bloodstream, clogging up our arteries, right? Wrong! Realize that quote came from 1985, and we now know that kind of thinking is simply old hat! (Or, perhaps I should say, given the topic, "old *fat!*") We know better now.

The cholesterol in your vessels doesn't just hang around. LDL knows that cholesterol is just waiting to be found! All this means is free cholesterol doesn't float around waiting to "gum up the works," adhering to blood vessels. The blood vessels are not even receptive to cholesterol in that form. As I've already taught you, in order to adhere to the endothelium, conditions have to be right, and part of that includes the presence of proinflammatory cytokines, adhesion molecules, and macrophages. The membrane also needs to be permeable, so there must be "endothelial activation," as we discussed. The LDL particles are there to scoop up blood cholesterol and integrate them into the lipoprotein structure to transport throughout the bloodstream.

Because, as I've shared with you already:

1) The cholesterol in the food you eat may have little to do with your ultimate total blood cholesterol level. That may have much more to do with your genetic predisposition.

2) Your total blood cholesterol is an inaccurate measure of heart attack risk. A more accurate measure is lipoprotein levels. **Lipoproteins** are a combination of a fat (**lipo-**) and a protein, and they function to package the types of fats (lipids)— including cholesterol, as well as triglycerides— from your food and other sources in your body and package them for transport through your bloodstream so they are soluble in your blood and carry them around to areas where they are needed. Why would they [lipids] be needed? Well, what you might not realize is that **cholesterol is necessary—indeed, vital—to life**. It is necessary to support the structural integrity of cell membranes. **Cholesterol is an essential precursor for the body to synthesize both male and female sex hormones.** It's even the substrate our body uses

to make Vitamin D! In fact, it just takes a couple of simple photochemical reactions to turn cholesterol into Vitamin D. **And if you don't have** *enough* **blood cholesterol, you could have a hemorrhagic stroke, among other deleterious health consequences.**

3) There are different classes of lipoproteins:

(a) **HDL**: also known as "good cholesterol." Not actually cholesterol, but **high-density lipoprotein.** Usually, when doctors talk about this value, we talk about HDL-C, which is that portion of cholesterol which is bound to high-density lipoprotein particles. If your doctor orders it, he or she can actually test for the number and size of HDL particles. This is more accurate, but also more expensive. Make sure you know the difference.

As you are probably aware, up until recently, most studies suggested that higher levels of HDL were protective against CVD (see below):

HDL Cholesterol level	Category
Less than 40 mg/dL	Heart disease risk
40-59 mg/dL	The higher, the better
Greater than 60 mg/dL	Protects against heart disease

However, very recently as of 2018, it has emerged that, like anything else, you can have "too much of a good thing," and very high levels of HDL, further, <u>certain subtypes of HDL may actually be harmful</u>. The most recent data seem to suggest that having very high HDL levels might not be as protective as we used to think and conversely low levels of HDL are not necessarily harmful. Certain subtypes of HDL found in patients with high HDL levels can actually worsen plaque buildup. Furthermore, certain patients with low total HDL levels seem to be protected from heart disease because even though they have low total HDL, they seem to have a higher percentage of the protective HDL

SUBTYPE. In my algorithm, The B-100 method, the subtypes of HDL are checked and their positive or negative impact on the risk of heart attack is calculated in order to come up with the correct heart attack prediction model.

(b) **LDL**: also known as "bad cholesterol." Again, not actually cholesterol, but **low-density lipoprotein**.

The recommended values of LDL that are published by the NIH are as follows:

LDL cholesterol level	Category
Less than 100 mg/dL	Optimal
100-129 mg/dL	Near optimal – above optimal
130-159 mg/dL	Borderline high
160-189 mg/dL	High
190 mg/dL and above	Very high

When doctors talk about LDL, we usually mean LDL-C, which is that portion of cholesterol bound to low-density lipoprotein particles. But LDL-C is not usually calculated directly. It is calculated according to what is called the Friedewald equation, which is not very exact. However, adding LDL-P, that is, a test for the size and number of LDL particles is more accurate and predictive than LDL-C alone.

(c) **VLDL: very-low-density lipoprotein**. Since VLDL also transports triglycerides and some cholesterol, it can be somewhat atherogenic as well, so it is important to keep levels of VLDL **under 40 mg/dL**.

A quick word about TRIGLYCERIDES as a risk factor for heart disease:

Triglycerides are a major constituent of body fat. They are made up of glycerol (which is a form of sugar) and three fatty acids. They allow the transfer of fat and blood glucose (sugar) to and from the liver from our fat tissues. Even though a triglyceride is a mix of fat and sugar, it is mostly categorized as fat and its level is checked with other cholesterol markers. It is however, mostly affected by carbohydrates and sugars we consume. Many studies have shown triglycerides to be a significant risk factor for the development of coronary artery disease. Unfortunately, most practitioners underestimate its risk. Also, most laboratories consider a fasting triglyceride levels of up to 150 mg/dl normal which is again unfortunate. An optimal fasting triglyceride level should be less than 100 mg/dl. (Triglyceride levels > 100 are associated with small dense LDL particles which, as we discussed above, are the most harmful form of LDL.)

Let's now go back to LDL.

Why is it better to test for LDL-P vs. just LDL-C?

There are actually a number of reasons for this, but the main reason is that current thinking among cardiologists is that CVD risk is better correlated with the number of LDL particles circulating in the bloodstream (LDL-P), rather than the amount of LDL cholesterol (LDL-C) carried within said particles (which, as I've alluded to earlier, may be rather inaccurate by calculation).

Another very good reason is that we are able to identify many discordant patients in whom LDL-P is elevated, but LDL-C is perfectly—and deceptively—normal. There is every reason to believe they are at increased risk of having a heart attack, and but for having an LDL-P test, we never would have caught it, and they could have slipped by undiagnosed, and had a heart attack.

In addition, we have been able to correlate genetic variations in the LDL receptor gene with Alzheimer's disease. So that's another test we can order.

Which only goes to show, again, it's not a cholesterol problem, it's a lipoprotein problem.

Yet, we have been told again and again, **"It's a cholesterol problem."** The AHA has said it for years. Our doctors, our parents, our teachers have said it. That's why we think: **we have to eat "low-fat, low-cholesterol diets to be heart-healthy."**

WHAT IF IT'S ALL AN ILLUSION?

For the last 60-plus years, conventional wisdom has held that saturated fat—the solid fat in meats, whole milk, cream, and butter—has been the artery-clogging culprit responsible for heart attacks. The basis for that theory started in the early 1950s, with the landmark Korean Soldiers Study, which examined autopsies performed on soldiers killed in action in the Korean War. The investigators were shocked to see 18- and 19-year-old boys who had developed significant coronary artery blockages that they did not expect to see on subjects that young. Upon microscopic examination, they noted their vessels were occluded with [what appeared to be] mostly saturated fat. And the fat "plaques" contained a good deal of cholesterol. From that study sprang the modern era of trying to control our dietary cholesterol.

Many a doctor and his patients have not found a simple, 1:1 correlation between the amount of cholesterol you eat (or saturated fat, which often contains a lot of cholesterol) and the amount of cholesterol you produce. Some patients, even if they eat relatively little cholesterol, have a genetic predisposition to produce a great deal of cholesterol, a condition which is called *familial hypercholesterolemia*. Patients with that condition can often have total cholesterol readings over 600 mg/dL. That is nothing to sneeze at, and we have to treat them with heavy-duty medication. Often, a statin alone is not sufficient for such patients to reduce their LDL-C into the normal range (New medications such as evolocumab—Repatha—are now available to significantly reduce their LDL-C level). [Due to such high cholesterol levels, these patients actually can have xanthomas, xanthelasmas, or yellowish, bumpy cholesterol deposits under their skin].

But, what about for less-extreme cases? As doctors, we were told to tell our patients for decades: Eat a low-fat, low-cholesterol diet to protect against atherosclerosis (those "fatty, cholesterol-filled plaques clogging your arteries"). Cut down on meats. Eat margarine instead of butter. Skim milk, or nonfat milk—never whole milk! These were the guidelines of the American Heart Association, and cardiologists like myself dutifully handed out the pamphlets. Those guidelines were based on decades of research, including the venerable Framingham Heart Study—probably one of the oldest continuing studies on heart health in existence. It started in 1948 and traced the health of people going back three generations.

**What if everything we thought we knew
about saturated fat was wrong?**
Two shocking studies suggest that may be true.

While I'm not suggesting the Framingham Study was a hack, every so often, investigators are brave enough to challenge such established dogma [ideas] as "saturated fats clog arteries" and test those assumptions anew. The PURE study, authored by Dr. Salim Yusuf, of McMaster University, followed 135,000 people from 18 different countries over a 7-year period. It showed that **high fat intake**—*whether total fat or saturated fat*—was associated with a **reduced** risk of mortality. Conversely, **high carbohydrate intake** was associated with an **increased** risk of mortality.[21] Another part of the study also found that eating 3-4 servings/day of fruits, vegetables, and legumes reduced mortality risk, with benefits increased if they were raw rather than cooked.[22]

If you look at the numbers, they tell the story. Here are the investigators' results:

---

21. Dehghan M, Mente A, Zhang X, et al. Associations of fats and carbohydrate intake with cardiovascular disease and mortality in 18 countries from five continents (PURE): A prospective cohort study Lancet 2017: DOI:10.1016/ S0140-6736(17)32252-3.
22. Miller V, Mente A, Dehghan M, et al. Fruit, vegetable, and legume intake, and cardiovascular disease and deaths in 18 countries (PURE): A prospective cohort study. Lancet 2017;DOI:10.1016/ S0140-6736(17)32253-5.

Hazard Ratio for Total Mortality (Highest Quintile vs Lowest Quintile)

Group	HR (95% CI)	P for trend
Carbohydrate	1.28 (1.12–1.46)	0.0001
Total fat	0.77 (0.67–0.87)	<0.0001
Saturated fat	0.86 (0.76–0.99)	0.0088
Monounsaturated fat	0.81 (0.71–0.92)	<0.0001
Polyunsaturated fat	0.80 (0.71–0.89)	<0.0001

For those of you who are intimidated by this chart, there is no reason to be.

"HR," or hazard ratio, just means the mortality rate of that group, compared to the control group, expressed as a ratio, with 1.00 being the same as the control group, or normal. Therefore, this data shows that the group eating more carbohydrates had a 1.28 times greater mortality rate than the control group, while the saturated fat group was only 86% as likely as the control group (-0.22 differential) to die.

The American Heart Association (AHA) is furious about this study, because their new advisory, released in 2017, recommends cutting saturated fat in favor of polyunsaturated fat and carbs. And, of course, replacing saturated fat with monounsaturated and polyunsaturated fats is what we cardiologists used to tell our patients as a matter of course. But now, here we have proof that saturated fat looks to be healthier than carbohydrates. But, it's just one study, right? It might be what we call an artifact. Not exactly! This study wasn't even the first one to assert the exact same blatantly in-your-face conclusion. Yes, it turns out the real bombshell exploded with this article, from the *British Journal of Sports Medicine*.[23] The title of the paper speaks for itself:

---

23. Malhotra A, Redberg RF, Meier P. Saturated fat does not clog the arteries: coronary heart disease is a chronic inflammatory condition, the risk of which can be effectively reduced from healthy lifestyle interventions. Br J Sports Med Published Online First: 25 April 2017. doi: 10.1136/bjsports-2016-097285

"Saturated fat does not clog the arteries: coronary heart disease is a chronic inflammatory condition, the risk of which can be effectively reduced from healthy lifestyle interventions."

The title of the article says it all, but the first paragraph is mind-blowing:

> *Coronary artery disease pathogenesis and treatment urgently requires a paradigm shift. Despite popular belief among doctors and the public, the conceptual model of dietary saturated fat clogging a pipe is just plain wrong. A landmark systematic review and meta-analysis of observational studies showed no association between saturated fat consumption and (1) all-cause mortality, (2) coronary heart disease (CHD), (3) CHD mortality, (4) ischemic stroke or (5) Type 2 diabetes in healthy adults.[24] Similarly in the secondary prevention of CHD there is no benefit from reduced fat, including saturated fat, on myocardial infarction, cardiovascular or all-cause mortality.[25] It is instructive to note that in an angiographic study of postmenopausal women with CHD, greater intake of saturated fat was associated with less progression[26] of atherosclerosis whereas carbohydrate and polyunsaturated fat intake were associated with greater progression.*

The reaction by AHA is predictable: Anyone who would contradict the well-rehearsed dictum of "saturated fat is the enemy" must, in their minds, therefore be the enemy. Think about it: The AHA has invested so much in that belief system,

24. de Souza RJ, Mente A, Maroleanu A, et al. Intake of saturated and trans-unsaturated fatty acids and risk of all-cause mortality, cardiovascular disease, and type 2 diabetes: systematic review and meta-analysis of observational studies. BMJ 2015;351:h3978.

25. Schwingshackl L, Hoffmann G. Dietary fatty acids in the secondary prevention of coronary heart disease: a systematic review, meta-analysis and meta-regression. BMJ Open 2014;4:e004487.

26. Mozaffarian D, Rimm EB, Herrington DM. Dietary fats, carbohydrate, and progression of coronary atherosclerosis in postmenopausal women. Am J Clin Nutr 2004;80:1175–84.

and it would feel pretty stupid admitting that it just might be wrong, but as President Reagan once said, "Facts are stupid things—stubborn things, I should say." He was saying that facts are stubborn because they stick—kind of like arterial plaque (which is made up of **oxidized-LDL-C**, right, boys and girls?). So, I think we, and the AHA, must give a really good listen.

But in the meantime, I would say enjoying that little pat of real, farm-fresh butter is OK.

A Bold Hypothesis: We have literally been *killing* ourselves with low-fat, low-cholesterol diets, when the problem was too much sugar, high-fructose corn syrup, and other refined carbs.

There has been considerable debate over the last several decades of whether "fat has been making us fat" or "carbs/sugar have been making us fat." (By the way, just in case anyone was wondering, yes, sugar is a carb—the prototypical, quintessential carb! Some people don't know... and that's OK!) Well, I now submit to you that that particular debate is now irrelevant, because what matters is our very survival. That's right. Which nutrient, fat (categorized by type) or carbohydrate, has the highest all-cause mortality rate? Somebody actually did that study. I just showed it to you above, and the answer is: carbs.

1. In our efforts to eat less fat and cholesterol, as a consequence, we naturally ate a great deal more carbs, both starches and sugars, to replace them on the plate. Not only that, we naturally crave sweet things, especially refined sugar and fructose.
2. The manufacturers of low-fat and low-cholesterol foods, in order to improve the taste profile of their processed food products, heavily boosted sugar content for us.
3. The truth of this assertion is proved by the endemic nature of metabolic syndrome/diabetes in this country.

The guidelines set forth by ACC/AHA (American College

of Cardiology/American Heart Association) prior to 2013 put the emphasis on cholesterol as the culprit for heart attack and cardiac mortality. It recommended treating every patient with high cholesterol levels with statins regardless of whether the patient had any risk factors for heart disease. For example, based on these guidelines, a healthy 20-year-old individual with moderately high cholesterol level, but with no other risk factors for heart disease, had to take statins for life!!

In 2013, the ACC/AHA came out with a revised set of recommendations. It recommended medical therapy with statins for four different cohort pools (people with a history of coronary artery disease, diabetics, people with LDL of >190 and patients with strong risk factors for heart disease). Anyone in any of these groups would automatically be put on statins and the dose of the statin increased to lower the LDL to <100 (or <70 in people with CAD).

Shortly after, the ACC/AHA again revised the guidelines and eliminated the target LDL goal. It recommended the HIGHEST dose of statins for the above group of patients and a moderate dose of statins for low-risk patients REGARDLESS of their cholesterol levels! Serious objections were raised by most practitioners. It seemed that guidelines were changing monthly. Furthermore, it caused too much confusion in regards to whom to put on statins and at what dose.

Finally, after almost two decades of going back and forth, the most recent guidelines published and presented in November of 2018 acknowledged the need for more personalization of the risk factors, and added a few more risk factors (presence of coronary calcium, chronic severe kidney disease, and postmenopausal status for women) before putting patients on statins. It also brought back the target goal for LDL cholesterol.

Even though finally, the new guidelines have definitely moved in the right direction, they still miss the root cause of coronary artery disease, and fail to address other major factors in the development of CAD. I am proud to say that none the patients under my care who have followed my method over more than a decade ago, have suffered a heart attack or died from it. That is because my program looks at all the underlying factors causing heart attack, not just simply cholesterol. My program is based on the assumption that it is not cholesterol that causes a heart attack, but rather what our body does to cholesterol that determines if someone eventually develops or dies of a heart attack.

Simply put, while everyone is an individual, there are way too many problems with the 2013 AHA/ACC guidelines, which represent the clinical standard of care for assessment and treatment of cardiovascular risk. Too many exceptions to the rule, such as discordant particle size-to-LDL-C patients; or patients who might have inflammatory markers, such as CRP, which would not ordinarily be screened for—or certainly, Lipoprotein(a), which we will discuss separately—would never be caught as risks for a heart attack under the current screening guidelines, because they might have completely run-of-the-mill total cholesterol, or LDL-C levels.

In my practice and my program, I consider 104 distinct variables, so nothing flies under the radar. If there's a biomarker that is well-studied and recognized, and we have investigated it, there's a good chance it's part of our battery of clinical tests.

The next chapter examines a very important risk factor for the development of coronary heart disease (CHD): INSULIN RESISTANCE and DIABETES: THE SUGAR LINK.

CHAPTER 5

THE SUGAR LINK

Sugar blues
Everybody's singin' the sugar blues
The whole town is ringin'
My lovin' man's sweet as can be
But the doggone fool's
Turned sour on me
I'm so unhappy
Feel so unhappy
I could lay me down and die
You could say what you choose
But I'm all confused
I got the sweet, sweet sugar blues
—More sugar!
I've got the sugar blues.

~ Ella Fitzgerald, **"Sugar Blues,"** Chick Webb & Ella Fitzgerald
Decca Sessions, © 1940, Decca Records.

Sugar in the morning
Sugar in the evening
Sugar at supper time
Be my little sugar and love me all the time.

~ The McGuire Sisters, **"Sugartime,"** (1958)

As I told you in the last chapter, the low-fat, low cholesterol crusaders, based on what they thought were the sound principles of the well-known Framingham Heart Study, by denying people the flavor inherent in fat, either naturally caused consumers to crave more sugar as a substitute for the fat, or caused manufacturers to systematically add more sugar to improve the flavor of their low-fat, low-cholesterol products, habituating the consumer to expect it in all of their foods—or a combination of both. The net effect was that the low-fat, low-cholesterol movement, rather than making us slim, trim, and heart-healthy, created a nation of dangerously-close-to-if-not-already-diabetic sugar addicts whose collective sweet tooth could never be satisfied. Worse, even though we were cutting fat, we were becoming a flabbier nation at severe risk of heart disease. The result seemed counterintuitive. What was going on? Well, as I said in the last chapter, I advanced the theory that carbs (of which sugar was the quintessential example) were making us fat, and I showed you a couple of studies with the surprising result that diets high in carbs led to greater all-cause mortality than diets high in saturated fat. What was not explained is why sugar is a putative risk factor for heart disease.

WHY IS SUGAR LINKED TO A GREATER RISK OF HEART DISEASE? WHAT'S THE CONNECTION?

Once again, inflammation of the blood vessels, specifically the vascular endothelium, is thought to be a factor. Not all the mechanisms are known, but consider the fact that diabetics have much higher rates of heart disease than the general population. As we discussed in the last chapter, diabetics suffer from two assaults on their vascular system: macrovascular and microvascular.

- **Macrovascular** disease refers to disease of the large blood vessels, especially the coronary arteries. A combination of high blood pressure and the deleterious effects of hyperglycemia (too much blood glucose)—in combination with endothelial dysfunction—sets the stage for atherosclerosis, and hence, oxidized LDL-containing plaque formation at the endothelium. When the plaques rupture, a heart attack or stroke results.

• **Microvascular** disease refers to disease of the smaller blood vessels, such as the peripheral arteries, notably those of the lower extremities. (The legs and feet are famous for being adversely affected in diabetes, and when proper care is not taken of them, tragic consequences can take place. How many of us have heard of, or know of people who are diabetic, who have had their limbs amputated?) Here, damage to blood vessels results from many years of exposure to overly high levels of blood glucose (hyperglycemia). The blood vessels react to this like an inflammatory/immune response. Also, glucose undergoes a series of *glycation* reactions, starting with the Maillard Reaction, which is the "browning" reaction that is responsible for the yummy taste of baked bread and browned meats. Unfortunately, it isn't so good for your body. The result for *you* is what is known as "advanced glycation end-products," or AGEs. These AGEs are now proven to cause the acceleration of diabetic complications, including diabetic cardiomyopathy (damage to the heart muscle), nephropathy (kidney damage), retinopathy (eye damage), and cataracts.

LANDMARK JAMA STUDY PROVES THE SUGAR LINK

Much of the how and why for the "sugar link" was mere conjecture—that is, until the publication of a very scary study in *JAMA*[27] (*Journal of the American Medical Association*) in 2014. The study's authors compared two groups of participants: one group consumed 10% of their daily calories from added sugar; the other group consumed 25% or more of their daily calories from added sugar. The investigators then followed them up for an average of 14.6 years and looked at how many in both groups died from cardiovascular disease (CVD). After adjusting for other factors, *the high-sugar group was 2.12 times as likely to die from CVD as the low-sugar group.* By the way,

---

27. Yang Q, Zhang Z. Added sugar intake and cardiovascular diseases mortality among US adults. JAMA Intern Med 2014; 174: 516–524.

the positive association between added sugar intake and CVD mortality remained significant even after the authors adjusted for conventional CVD risk factors, such as blood pressure and total cholesterol. The association they observed between the percentage of calories consumed from added sugar and increased risk of CVD mortality was largely consistent across age group, sex, race/ethnicity (except among non-Hispanic blacks), as well as educational attainment, physical activity level, and BMI. Why was this?

SOME POSSIBLE EXPLANATIONS/MECHANISMS

1) **Added Sugars Drive Insulin Resistance/Hyperinsulinemia**
   A recent article advanced the theory that many people who have CVD, or heart attacks, may be suffering from hyperglycemia (elevated blood glucose) but simply not know it, or have any symptoms of it.[28] This study illuminated a stunning fact, namely, that according to another study they found, *nearly three-quarters of patients who showed up in the hospital with an acute myocardial infarction ("MI" – otherwise known as a heart attack) have abnormal glucose tolerance, and fully half have diabetes.*[29] Six months after their heart attack, 43% of these patients *still* had abnormal glucose tolerance, which is approximately three times higher than that found in matched controls (15%). Therefore, this data appears to demonstrate that high blood glucose does not appear to be merely a temporary or short-term finding in patients who have suffered a heart attack, because many of these patients have continued to have abnormal glucose tolerance even when they are followed for a number of years after the initial heart attack.

---

28. DiNicolantonio JJ, OKeefe JH. Added sugars drive coronary heart disease via insulin resistance and hyperinsulinemia: a new paradigm. Open Heart 2017;4:e000729.
29. Sowton E. Cardiac infarction and the glucose-tolerance test. Br Med J 1962; 1:84–6.

What do we mean by insulin resistance, and how does it work?

Insulin is, of course, a hormone produced by the beta cells of the pancreas, which functions to "mop up" excess glucose in the blood. Glucose is not ingested most of the time but made in the liver by splitting disaccharides like sucrose. Characteristics of insulin resistance are:

(a) When the cells of the body fail to respond to insulin normally, *blood glucose levels remain high and hyperglycemia results.* This is termed "insulin resistance" or "abnormal glucose tolerance."

(b) **This condition prompts the pancreas to produce more insulin.** Insulin is, although many of us don't consider it as such, a growth factor. And it is very good at promoting fat synthesis in the body, a process called lipogenesis. Lipogenesis occurs in both fatty tissue, called adipocytes, and liver cells, known as hepatocytes. In either of these places (adipose tissue or liver), insulin is equally potent at binding to insulin receptors, and stimulating lipogenesis.

In patients eating diets that are carbohydrate-rich, lipogenesis is stimulated. Conversely, in patients with diets high in polyunsaturated fatty acids (PUFA), lipogenesis is decreased.

(c) Now, thanks to the excess insulin production, you have produced a *bunch of fatty tissue, which is naturally much more resistant to the insulin.*[30]

(d) Eating a diet high in added sugars, especially fructose, is known to increase insulin resistance. This is why you may have heard people getting upset about manufacturers using *high fructose corn syrup* in sodas.

(e) Excess blood insulin levels alone (hyperinsulinemia) have been demonstrated to be an *independent* risk factor for coronary heart disease (CHD).

30. Bruckdorfer, KR; Kang, SS; Yudkin, J; (1974) Insulin sensitivity of adipose tissue of rats fed with various carbohydrates. Proc Nutr Soc, 33 (1) 4A-5A.

(f) Therefore, both human and animal data strongly indicate that *the overconsumption of added sugars— both sucrose and fructose—drives insulin resistance and hyperinsulinemia, and thus CVD mortality risk.*

(g) Unlike most other tissues in our body, a healthy heart uses fatty acids for energy and to function. *During a heart attack, the heart throws its ordinary energy source of free fatty acids right out the window for a sugar fix.* Or, to put it another way, the heart knows what the heart wants ... and it wants glucose. It's sweet, it burns quickly, gets the job done, and has tons of energy? If you were your heart, would you blame it? You just had a heart attack. Would a bunch of heavy, greasy, high-molecular-weight, so-called *"free"* fatty acids really sound that appetizing to you under the circumstances? Uh-uh. We didn't think so either. So, because of that trade-off, if you have insulin resistance or diabetes already, your chances of surviving that heart attack are already going to be lower because you will be less likely to be able to supply your heart with that quick glucose source (because, remember, insulin helps transport that glucose and that function is not working so well if you have insulin resistance!)

Also, diets high in added sugar are known to increase your chances of developing diabetes as well as insulin resistance. The study authors hypothesize that this may well lead to larger MIs (myocardial infarctions), which portend a higher risk of CHD mortality, a bold statement.

2) Added Sugars Drive an Inflammatory Cascade.

Even in the absence of causing diabetes, the above-referenced paper showed that people who ate diets high in added sugars consistently suffered a higher number of deleterious cardiac events by causing heightened glucose tolerance. Other investigators have posited that this means that the continuing interaction between high levels of blood glucose and the vascular endothelium is the first step of an inflammatory cascade which ultimately results in the formation of an atheroma (a lesion of an atherosclerotic plaque). Another group of researchers[31] suggests that insulin resistance in adipose tissue (which I described earlier), sets off the inflammatory cascade by recruitment of monocytes to what is known as visceral white adipose tissue (think of that deep, central belly fat). Then the monocytes differentiate into proinflammatory M1 macrophages.

3) Added Sugar, Especially Fructose, Increases Hypertension (High Blood Pressure).

As if all of the foregoing weren't enough to convince you of the data linking sugar to CVD, there is actually experimental data now showing that eating—or rather, drinking—sugar, in the form of sugary soft drinks, increases hypertension (high blood pressure).[32] And, as you know, high blood pressure is a component of metabolic syndrome, and also increases your chance of dying from CVD (heart attack or stroke). It also turns out that fructose is much worse than sucrose for you in causing high blood pressure, and there was apparently reason for concern about the addition of high fructose corn syrup to cola and soda products.[33, 34]

INSULIN RESISTANCE VS. DIABETES AND CORONARY DISEASE

By now, it should be very clear that diabetes is the most important

31. Shimobayashi M, Albert V, Woelnerhanssen B. Insulin resistance causes inflammation in adipose tissue. J Clin Invest. 2018;128(4):1538-1550.
32. DiNicolantonio JJ, Lucan SC. The wrong white crystals: not salt but sugar as aetiological in hypertension and cardiometabolic disease. Open Heart 2014;1:e000167.
33. Brown CM, Dulloo AG, Yepuri G, Montani JP. Fructose ingestion acutely elevates blood pressure in healthy young humans. Am J Physiol Regul Integr Comp Physiol. 2008 Mar;294(3):R730-7. Epub 2008 Jan 16.
34. Malik VS, Popkin BM, Bray GA, Després J-P, Hu FB. Sugar Sweetened Beverages, Obesity, Type 2 Diabetes and Cardiovascular Disease Risk. Circulation. 2010;121(11):1356-1364.

risk factor for coronary artery disease, heart attack, and cardiac death. However, what most people, including physicians, cardiologists and endocrinologists and practitioners who consider themselves diabetologists either don't know or report is that the process of atherosclerosis or plaque buildup in the coronary arteries start way before most people consider themselves diabetic or even Pre-diabetic. This is a very important point which we emphasize greatly in our clinics and to our patients.

If you are determined to be insulin dependent, you already have dysfunctional coronary endothelium and your arteries are busy building plaques. This is why, in my B-100 algorithm, diabetes and insulin resistance almost have the same weight. Patients in our B-100 programs are treated aggressively to reverse the insulin resistance.

CHAPTER 6

THE GUT MICROBIOTA

Did you know more than **half** of your body is not human? Your own cells make up only 43% of your body's total cell count. The rest are microscopic colonists. These microscopic colonists are overwhelmingly bacteria and half of them reside in your gut. The bacteria in your gut are enough to fill a large can of soup, about 5 lbs! We now know these "good" bacteria are responsible for keeping you emotionally and physically healthy. Conversely, the lack of these "good bacteria" can attribute to diseases ranging from depression and mental health issues to immune and autoimmune conditions to all types of gastrointestinal symptoms and yes, we now know that they can lead to heart and cardiovascular disease including heart attacks (as we shall see later in the chapter). It is the natural variations between individual bacteria in our gut that make one susceptible to certain diseases and some others immune from ever getting them.

THE "GASTROINTESTINAL MICROBIOME"
— *I just got a feeling in the pit of my stomach.*

For so many of my patients, when they have been asked to recall what preceded any descriptions of general malaise, invariably, the answer has been gastrointestinal in nature when they are discussing what symptoms preceded the "presenting complaint." but first let's discuss the difference between the "**microbiome**" and the "**microbiota**?" *Is* there even one? Is the *microbiota* just a more Sci-Fi sounding name? ('cause it definitely *sounds* like Sci-Fi stuff.)

The easiest way to think about it is: The human **microbiota** is like the whole universe of microorganisms (microbes) that your body plays host to, including bacteria, viruses, and other single-celled critters. The overwhelming majority of these microbes reside in the comfortable environment of the gut. Hence, we are now referring to the *gut microbiota*. The genetic material (genes, DNA, RNA, etc.) contained within the gut microbiota is the gut **microbiome**. Now that you have the definitions down, why are they so important, anyway? Why should we care so much about these things? Because, guess what, folks? When it comes right down to it, some of the most important things in our lives— **including our cardiovascular system**—are controlled, indeed, tightly regulated by our gut microbiomes. For those of you who think this is somehow a newfangled fad, it really isn't. The signs were there, and for those who cared to learn, the microbes presented a classic lesson for the annals of medicine:

"Don't Stress Yourself Out! You're Gonna Give Yourself an Ulcer!"

How many times have we heard someone (even ourselves) say these words? Where did they come from? Well, they came from the idea that too much stress, in addition to an excess of stomach acid, and overly-spicy food, was the cause of peptic ulcer. Why? Because this was simply common knowledge. That's why our medicine cabinets regularly are stocked with Tums and Rolaids, isn't it? You know, you're just going to give yourself added stress, and that, my friend—you guessed it—may just give you an *ulcer*!

Cut to 1982. A defiant young doctor, Barry Marshall, M.D., was, slowly but surely, becoming a rock star!

AN ACID-LOVING BACTERIUM

Dr. Marshall, along with his co-investigator, Robin Warren, started sampling the stomach fluids of his patients who had gastritis and peptic ulcer and he noticed that they had spiral-shaped bacteria,[35] which he cultured. When he submitted the data for publication, their reception was chilly, and most journals refused to publish his results. Their argument was that no bacteria could *possibly* survive under the acidic conditions of the stomach (which produces hydrochloric acid), so they simply rejected the data as nonsense.

In fact, in 1983, Drs. Marshall and Warren submitted their findings to the Gastroenterological Society of Australia, but the reviewers turned their paper down; not only that, but they rated it in the bottom 10% of the papers they'd received that year. But, as a very famous person once said, "nevertheless, he persisted." Why? Well, Dr. Marshall himself offers perhaps the most compelling reason: "Everyone was against me, but I knew I was right."[36] We now know there are certain types of bacteria that actually thrive under acidic conditions, and the one that Dr. Marshall discovered is one classic example: *Helicobacter pylori.* If that name sounds familiar to you, it should: That's because *H. pylori* is now universally acknowledged as a major causative agent of peptic ulcer disease.

"PUBLISH…OR PERISH?"

There is an old cliché in the academic world called "publish or perish," which means, you'd better *publish* your studies, get your name out there, or else you'll perish, because someone else will publish their works first and beat you to the punch.

---

35. Marshall, B.J., et al. Unidentified Curved Bacilli in The Stomach of Patients with Gastritis and Peptic Ulceration, The Lancet , Volume 323 , Issue 8390 , 1311 – 1315.
36. "Barry Marshall Interview, H. Pylori and the Making of a Myth." Academy of Achievement. 23 May 1998

But, in Dr. Marshall's case, perhaps he took the saying a *bit* too literally: He was extremely frustrated by the rejection letters of the scientific journals. Not just from a personal standpoint, but professionally as well, because he felt that he, and other colleagues, would be able to have patients that would be able to benefit from this data being published. Dr. Marshall was hamstrung by the fact that he was unable to duplicate the results by infecting pigs and mice with the bacterium, because *H. pylori* is essentially based in primates, and so it does not like to grow in pigs or mice.

HIS OWN GUINEA PIG

Wanting to prove his case to the world, and show he just **knew he was right, Dr. Marshall did the logical thing: He drank a broth filled with millions of *H. pylori* organisms**—hey, why not!—**and consequently, infected himself!**

CONNECTING THE DOTS: H. PYLORI, ULCERS, AND CANCER, OH MY!

Ultimately, Drs. Marshall and Warren were able to prove that *H. pylori* was inextricably linked to ulcers and inflammation, both of which are linked to stomach cancer. Their discovery has taught us the importance of the gut microbiome (just by the illustration of one microorganism here) and how it can affect the development of inflammation and cancer, as well as other diseases.

EXTRAPOLATING THE KNOWLEDGE

We know that certain microorganisms that we have seen in colonies are beneficial, such as L. acidophilus., and that's why we include them in probiotic formulas. On the other hand, certain bacterial strains are considered undesirable because their presence is correlated with higher levels of oxidative stress, as well as higher levels of inflammatory biomarkers. Your gut flora also *changes with age.* For example, *Proteobacteria* predominates in the gut of newborns but is then substantially reduced from that age ($\approx16\%$) to adulthood ($\approx4.6\%$) (Gritz et al., 2015). And, a bad diet may further negatively impact your gut microbiome "New Age" foods rich in calories with reduced fiber, facilitate the aberrant expansion of *Proteobacteria*—which you can find in both inflammatory bowel disease (IBD) and metabolic disorders (Wilson et al., 2016; Wilson et al., 2015). Particularly, an increased *Firmicutes/Bacteroidetes* ratio has been found to be associated with a high risk of CVD (Abdallah Ismail et al., 2011).

However, simply adding the well-known probiotic *Bifidobacterium animalis* treatment improved insulin sensitivity. Thus, this demonstrated that the probiotic intervention could reverse a high-fat-diet-(HFD)-induced adverse metabolic phenotype (Amar et al., 2011). This association was further strengthened by a study in which the mice who were fed with both an HFD and *Akkermansia muciniphila* were protected from developing insulin resistance, demonstrated improved gut integrity, and exhibited less tissue inflammation compared to those fed with an HFD alone.

These are very powerful initial studies. The research in the field of microbiomes has exploded over the past three years as we have learned and continue to learn the relationship between our gut microbiomes and our disease states. There are many centers now that offer "fecal transplant" with surprisingly great results! (I am not advocating or rejecting this therapy – we still need to know more about it. I am not at present recommending or rejecting it in my proactive). However, stool testing is an important part of my integrative approach to determine the health of our patient's gut which affects the patient's cardiovascular system.

Furthermore, I recommend a specific form of probiotic for my patient as a way to improve and protect their cardiovascular health. We are currently conducting experiments on newer and more effective strains of the probiotic and it is my hope that as an integrative and preventive cardiologist, I will soon be able to give my patients other proactive medical therapies that include bacterial infusions that may repopulate the gut. These therapies will not only strengthen the immune system and make it more resistant to infections, but they will also reduce the chances of coronary atherosclerosis and heart disease.

THE GUT MICROBIOME, RED MEAT AND "TMAO" A MARKER FOR HEART DISEASE

(This Is Why Red Meat Is "So Bad for You?")

Gut bacteria could cause cardiovascular disease by influencing appetite, fat creation and insulin sensitivity. However, a more important mechanism involves how we digest two key nutrients: choline and L-carnitine. Choline is abundant in animal cell membranes, egg yolk and high-fat dairy products; L-carnitine is found mostly in red meat. Unfortunately, they are also marketed as nutritional supplements, with L-carnitine being a frequent ingredient in energy drinks. **When dietary choline and L-carnitine come in contact with certain <u>bacteria in the intestine</u>, they are metabolized into TMA.** One of the huge outgrowths of all the recent research on the gut microbiome was the discovery of TMA. Haven't heard of it? I guess you're just not one of the cool people like me. But all joking aside, you will hear about it soon. It actually has been the subject of articles in the mainstream media. TMA stands for trimethylamine.

Once the gut bacteria produces TMA, it makes its way to the liver, where an enzyme converts it to TMAO (trimethylamine-*N*-oxide). TMAO ends up in the bloodstream, where it affects the whole-body cholesterol metabolism, vascular inflammation and formation of unstable plaques in the arterial walls.

There is a veritable litany of studies casting TMAO in the role of malefactor, linking it to heart attack and heart failure,[37, 38] as well as the metabolic syndrome, and inflammation, obesity, and atherosclerosis. In one experimental study, adding choline, carnitine, pre-carnitine or even TMAO alone to the diet, was sufficient to enhance macrophage cholesterol load and atherosclerotic plaque formation.[39]

THE RED MEAT CONNECTION

Even the name of the amino acid *carnitine* is charged, revealing its meaty origins, and the test results involving it do not contradict the expectations. Van Hecke and colleagues studied the effect of white vs. red meat consumption on oxidative stress, TMAO, and inflammation in Sprague-Dawley rats. Compared to the chicken diets, consumption of the beef diets resulted in higher urinary trimethylamine (4.5-fold) and TMAO (3.7-fold) concentrations. Also, rats on the fat beef diet had higher renal MDA (+24.4%) and heart MDA (+12.9%) and lower liver vitamin E (-26.2%) compared to all other diets such as lean beef, lean chicken diets (Van Hecke et al., 2016). So as much as the "meat-and-potatoes men" among us might have wished for a different result, those numbers are a bit frightening. Also, the increased plasma TMAO level was associated with the increased TNF-α, IL-6 and C-reactive protein —all of which are inflammatory biomarkers!

These results, taken together, suggest we should seriously

37. Tang WH, Wang Z, Shrestha K, Borowski AG, Wu Y, Troughton RW, *et al.* (2015b). Intestinal microbiota-dependent phosphatidylcholine metabolites, diastolic dysfunction, and adverse clinical outcomes in chronic systolic heart failure. *Journal of cardiac failure* **21**(2): 91-96.
38. Troseid M, Ueland T, Hov JR, Svardal A, Gregersen I, Dahl CP, *et al.* (2015). Microbiota-dependent metabolite trimethylamine-N-oxide is associated with disease severity and survival of patients with chronic heart failure. *Journal of internal medicine* **277**(6): 717-726.
39. Koeth RA, Levison BS, Culley MK, Buffa JA, Wang Z, Gregory JC, *et al.* (2014). gamma-Butyrobetaine is a proatherogenic intermediate in gut microbial metabolism of L-carnitine to TMAO. *Cell metabolism* **20**(5): 799-812.

consider looking into some probiotics (and my team is always at the forefront of examining new ones) as well as cutting down on red meat, dairy and excessive egg yolk consumption.

CHAPTER 7

HEAVY METAL TOXICITY

While I'm sure my patients of a certain age will say that they just knew that listening to all those Black Sabbath records couldn't have been good for you, professionals in my line of work know there's a difference between those types of Heavy Metal and what I am talking about here. When I say, "heavy metal toxicity," I literally mean toxicity [to your cardiovascular system] caused by "heavy metals," as in lead, arsenic, cadmium, mercury, and cobalt.

Now, it may seem obvious that the aforementioned metals (e.g., what constitutes "heavy" is usually based on atomic weight on the periodic table, density, and chemical properties) would be considered toxic, but mainstream medicine never really dealt with the topic, except in the context of forensics (when we were looking at autopsy results to see whether somebody was poisoned to death), and complementary/integrative medicine's approach, which proposed widespread testing for heavy metal exposure, followed by chelation therapy, which was considered impractical, and too expensive. What's more, an entire industry sprang up around removing amalgam fillings due to their mercury content, but without even testing blood levels first.

However, what we know today, and what I apply in my practice, is grounded in evidence-based medicine, not hype. And the evidence has traditional, old-school cardiologists scratching their heads, questioning everything. Yet, the study results (from a study called TACT—Trial to Assess Chelation Therapy[40]) were telling a different story. A study that they, the *Establishment* cardiologists, had only approved because they were sure it would debunk chelation as a fraud and a myth once and for all. This wasn't supposed to happen, and yet, it was happening, despite all odds. It was a completely unexpected result. But, amazingly enough, it did. Like with everything else I've taught you, you must understand how we got here.

In 2002, a group of ACAM (American College for Advancement of Medicine) physicians who were using chelation in their own practices, or believed in the technique, to treat atherosclerotic heart disease, were looking to do a clinical study in order to prove its effectiveness once and for all. At the same time, a group of traditional physicians felt that the ACAM practitioners performing chelation treatments were selling false hope to desperate patients; they believed there was no possibility that chelation could offer any benefit to patients with cardiovascular disease (CVD). Therefore, they were eager to work together with the ACAM physicians to help them get their clinical study set up and funded.

This study was called TACT—Trial to Assess Chelation Therapy. However, they were trying to debunk chelation as a legitimate medical treatment, and hoped that, by doing the study, they would be able to get the results to prove, once and for all, that it was the fraud they all knew it was—and was probably dangerous to patients to boot. They took 1,708 patients for the study, all of whom were over 50 years old, and had had a prior heart attack, and divided them randomly into two groups: half would get the chelation treatment with a substance called disodium EDTA (ethylenediamine tetraacetic acid)—some of which had vitamins added, some didn't; the other half, a saline placebo. They had 40 IV infusions over nearly a year.

---

40. Lamas GA, Goertz C, Boineau R, et al. TACT Investigators. Effect of disodium EDTA chelation regimen on cardiovascular events in patients with previous myocardial infarction: the TACT randomized trial. JAMA. 2013;309:1241–1250.

On November 4, 2012, the American Heart Association held its annual meeting in Los Angeles, and the investigators from the TACT trial had done their follow-ups, analyzed the data, and now, were releasing their results to the audience. Those results were shocking: The EDTA infusion group had achieved an 18% reduction in all types of "heart events" (defined as death, another heart attack, stroke, stenting or bypass, and hospitalization for heart pains) over and above that provided by standard treatment with statins and aspirin.[41] The (EDTA plus vitamins) infusion group did even better: Their heart events were reduced by 26% when compared to placebo.[40] And, to top it all off, the study patients who were diabetic had a response that could be deemed nothing less than dramatic: they experienced "a 41% reduction in clinical events," which included a 43% decrease in deaths over a 5-year period. As the authors put it, "There is nothing comparable in diabetes therapies."[42]

The foregoing results were actually so unexpected that, rather than the audience being impressed at these ground-breaking results, many participants in the audience, as well as the cardiology community at large greeted the results either with skepticism ("this is *probably* wrong") or downright disbelief ("this is *definitely* wrong and cannot possibly be right").[43] Nearly everyone involved, including several of the investigators, were expecting a negative result. The actual results were even described as an "embarrassment" for many of the people involved in the trials because, remember, these results indicated that chelation therapy—something most of the cardiology community thought was snake oil—not only *worked*, but had an additive effect

41. Lamas G, Boineau R, Goertz C, et al. EDTA Chelation Therapy Alone and in Combination with Oral High-Dose Multivitamins and Minerals for Coronary Disease: The Factorial Group Results of the Trial to Assess Chelation Therapy. Am Heart J. 2014;168:37–44.
42. Escolar E, Lamas G, Mark DB, et al. The Effect of an EDTA-based Chelation Regimen on Patients with Diabetes and Prior Myocardial Infarction in TACT. Circ Cardiovasc Qual Outcomes. 2014;7:15–24.
43. Kaiser C. AHA: Dismay Greets Positive Chelation Study.[Accessed May 10, 2018];MedPage Today. 2012 Nov.4; Available at: http://www.medpagetoday.com/MeetingCoverage/AHA/35746.

in protecting against new cardiac events as compared to the standard, first-line pharmaceutical therapies that cardiologists have been prescribing for years, i.e., statins and aspirin, especially in diabetic patients, to a huge degree.

Another problem for mainstream cardiologists was that they claimed that they could not explain a feasible mechanism for EDTA chelation and therefore, there was no way they could feel comfortable with the results that they were seeing from the TACT trial. The investigators behind TACT are looking to validate and replicate the results of TACT with a new study, called TACT2, which is currently underway. That should help people feel more comfortable. However, medicine has provided us with many examples where we did not originally know the mechanism of action of certain drugs, but we simply discovered they worked by accident. The use of sildenafil citrate (Viagra) for erectile dysfunction—originally developed for high blood pressure and angina—and thalidomide to treat leukemia and multiple myeloma—originally developed to treat morning sickness in women, to great catastrophe in the 1950s—are but two prominent examples of serendipity.[44]

As an integrative cardiologist, I have been looking at the data on chelation therapy for many years, and it just makes sense, because it's just basic biochemistry—nothing newfangled or "alternative" there. First, you need to understand what chelation is all about.

WHAT IS CHELATION?

Chelation (key-LAY-shun) comes from a Greek word meaning "claw," which may be helpful for you to visualize. Think of the "claw games" you used to play at arcades as kids to win prizes. That's what chelating agents, like EDTA, are kind of like. They are like big claws, or teeth. In fact, chelating agents are

---

44. Lamas GA, Navas-Acien A, Mark DB, Lee KL. Heavy Metals, Cardiovascular Disease, and the Unexpected Benefits of Edetate Disodium Chelation Therapy. J Am. Coll. Cardiol. 2016;67(20):2411-2418.

called *dentate ligands* based on the fact that they have "teeth," or places to bind to their targets, which are **metals**. EDTA is a *hexa*dentate ligand because it is a claw-shaped molecule with six "teeth," so it can wrap around a metal ion very effectively. It's a real metalmouth!

Back in Germany, in 1938, a man named Munz patented ethylenediamine tetraacetic acid (EDTA) as a substitute for citric acid in order to sequester calcium from hard water to prevent it from causing stains in textile printing. During World War I, a great deal of poison gas was used, and antidotes were later developed in the '30s and '40s in order to try to deal with poison gas injuries and thus try to reduce the casualties that happened on the battlefield. Some of the antidotes, such as BAL (British Anti-Lewisite), worked by chelation: BAL, or dimercaprol, functioned as a bidentate ligand, and chelated the heavy metal arsenic in the poison gas Lewisite. Unfortunately, it, too, was quite toxic. Somewhere along the way, people working on EDTA figured out that it chelated lead very effectively, and there were multiple clinical reports of the calcium disodium salt of EDTA being used this way.[45]

EDTA CLEANS CALCIFIED ARTERIES IN 1956 ... AND NOBODY REMEMBERS

Then, in 1956, Clarke, et al. wrote a paper of historic proportions: It was the first paper ever to use IV infusions of disodium ethylenediamine tetraacetate (a.k.a. disodium edetate) to treat atherosclerotic heart disease, and it reported improvement in an astonishing 19 out of 20 patients with angina.[46] The authors noted that it required about 20 infusions in order for this improvement to become evident. Keep in mind, back in 1956, there were no effective treatments for CVD, there were no statins or stents, and

45. Rubin M, Gignac S, Bessman SP, et al. Enhancement of lead excretion in humans by disodium calcium ethylene-diamine tetraacetate. Science. 1953;117:659–660
46. Clarke CN, Clarke NE, Mosher RE. Treatment of angina pectoris with disodium ethylene diamine tetraacetic acid. Am J Med Sci. 1956;232:654–666.

although aspirin was around, people didn't know to take it to prevent heart attacks. Cigarette smoking was not thought to cause atherosclerosis; and a goodly proportion of doctors smoked!

However, the investigators were struck by the fact that the hearts that they saw in autopsies revealed significantly-calcified coronary arteries. From this simple observation, Clarke and his collaborators reasoned that perhaps the disodium edetate was decalcifying coronary obstructions within the arteries, and thereby relieving his study subjects' angina. After all, recall that the initial patent application for EDTA was as a *calcium* chelator. This study, one would think, would have made front-page news, and started a trend, but of course, it didn't. There was one small study in 1963, which was deemed "a reappraisal," but did not control for other risk factors.[47] Therefore, the advent of the Swingin' Sixties, which brought a raft of new approaches to treating CVD, most of which were surgical—don't forget, this was the decade that made stars of Dr. Christiaan Barnard and Dr. Michael DeBakey, and blocked arteries could simply be bypassed—and what wasn't surgical was chemical. (There were cholesterol-lowering drugs before statins, such as cholestyramine resin, and the whole problem was thought to be cholesterol, remember?) Therefore, a cumbersome treatment like a 20-plus series of IV infusions was quickly forgotten.

What TACT has shown us—and what the new TACT2 trial will hopefully show us—is that this method of clearing calcium from the blood vessels of 62 years ago still holds true. However, there is much more to it. It's something that many of us have not come to grips with, unfortunately.

It was something that was originally dismissed as solely the province of "alternative" or "complementary" physicians. Now, because I am an integrative cardiologist, it is something I have been *integrating* into my practice because it has, unfortunately, become part of my knowledge base: the realization that heavy

---

47. Kitchell JR, Palmon F, Jr, Aytan N, et al. The treatment of coronary artery disease with disodium EDTA. A reappraisal. Am J Cardiol. 1963;11:501–506.

metals, over the years, have accumulated in our bodies, and contributed to our overall cardiac risk.

"Don't You Know That You're Toxic?"

You're toxic, I'm slippin' under
With a taste of a poison paradise
I'm addicted to you
Don't you know that you're toxic?
And I love what you do
Don't you know that you're toxic?
Too high, can't come down
It's in the air and it's all around.

~ Britney Spears, "Toxic," *In the Zone* (2003)

"IT'S IN THE AIR AND IT'S ALL AROUND"

First of all, I think I can safely say I believe no other cardiology book has ever quoted a Britney Spears song. But there is wisdom in the words of Britney: *you* are indeed toxic. Maybe not the way she was referring to in the song, but you are, and have been rendered so by your body's accumulation of toxic elements—heavy metals—which are in the air and are all around. As consumers of the modern age, most of us are addicted to the "poison paradise" of convenience that has been created for us, even knowing that we have been made toxic by it. Now, I defy any of my dear readers and patients to do that kind of deconstructionist analysis on a Britney lyric of your choice in the context of another modern medical problem. Try it sometime: it's fun and will amaze your friends.

But seriously, folks. How did we get to be so toxic?

LEAD

Those of you who were a certain age will remember going to the gas station and the attendant (yes, they had those at one time) asking you, "Regular, or Ethyl?" Well, "Ethyl" meant tetraethyl lead, which was an anti-knock compound added to gasoline up until approximately 1988 (even later in some places), before everybody was required to switch to unleaded gasoline. Although it's hard to believe now, most people had used leaded gas. This is the source of most of the lead in your bodies if you are old enough to have been exposed in that manner. Then, there is lead paint, which was widely applied up through the '70s, and could easily chip off, and which kids could be exposed to in a variety of ways. Lead acetate was even used in Grecian Formula hair dye. We simply did not have any idea how bad lead was back then in small doses when you were not being "poisoned." Yet, now we know the cardiovascular consequences it has, and they are downright scary.

For example, in a recent study that examined the blood and bone levels of lead in a group of 868 men, the investigators broke down the subjects into three groups (tertiles): the first with bone levels of less than 22 micrograms of lead in their patellas (knee bones); the second tertile, between 22 and 35 micrograms of lead, and the third, over 35 micrograms. The group in the highest tertile had a 5.63 times greater risk of death from cardiovascular causes and an 8.37 times greater risk of death from ischemic heart disease specifically than those in the lowest tertile (those who had the least lead in their knee bones).[48] Not only is lead toxic per se, it actually raises your blood pressure. This effect is well known.[49,50] Ironically, that rise in blood pressure you'll be getting from all that lead will be measured in—what else, millimeters of that great other toxic metal—mercury!

48. Weisskopf MG, Jain N, Nie H, Sparrow D, Vokonas P, Schwartz J, et al.
A prospective study of bone lead concentration and death from all causes, cardiovascular diseases, and cancer in the Department of Veterans Affairs Normative Aging Study. Circulation. 2009;120(12):1056–1064.
49. Harlan WR, Landis JR, Schmouder RL, Goldstein NG, Harlan LC
Blood lead, blood pressure. Relationship in the adolescent and adult US population. JAMA: Journal of the American Medical Association. 1985;253(4):530–534.
50. Pirkle JL, Schwartz J, Landis JR, Harlan WR. The relationship between blood lead levels and blood pressure and its cardiovascular risk implications. American Journal of Epidemiology. 1985;121(2):246–258.

MERCURY

The U.S. Government has ranked mercury as the third most toxic environmental hazard after arsenic and lead.[51] Although we are usually aware of "silver" fillings possibly containing mercury amalgam (not all of them do), there are less obvious sources. You may not realize it if you live near mercury mining sites, recycling facilities, medical or municipal incinerators, coal-fired power plants, or have been exposed to mercury-containing latex paint.[52] And if you have been trying to eat right by eating less red meat by stocking up on fish, you may have been inadvertently poisoning yourself in the process, since many fish are contaminated with mercury. The relative risk of cardiovascular death from high mercury levels appears to be significantly higher—although high fish intake does seem to be a confounding factor, because of the healthy fish oil! But I wouldn't try to tempt fate. The risk of the mercury still outweighs the omega-3's and DHA.

ARSENIC

This goes without saying, I would think. You know arsenic is really bad. It's a straight-up poison! If you've seen any murder mysteries, you know this. Interestingly enough, we used to use arsenic in medicine to treat certain diseases, and it saved lives. These medicines were called arsenicals. In fact, there are still a couple of them in use today: one is arsenic trioxide, which is an inorganic arsenical, and another one is a derivative of it called darinaparsin, or S-dimethylarsino-glutathione, which is an organic version. These are incredibly toxic compounds, and they are used to fight lymphomas. The idea being that—as with most chemotherapy—you have to use something toxic in hopes

---

51. Agency for Toxic Substances and Disease Registry (ATSDR) The priority list of hazardous substances. Atlanta (GA): U.S. Department of Health and Human Services, Public Health Service; 2011.
52. Berlin M, Zalups RK, Fowler BA. In: Mercury. Third Edition. Nordberg GF, Fowler BA, Nordberg M, Friberg LT, editors. Elsevier: Handbook on the Toxicology of Metals; 2007. pp. 675–729.

of killing the cancer cell. And, like many chemotherapy drugs, they are probably cardiotoxic. Just handling these compounds requires gloves and special equipment. But, back to arsenic.

HOW, AND WHERE, ARE WE NORMALLY EXPOSED TO ARSENIC?

This ain't chicken feed. Or actually, it probably is! Chicken feed used to contain a compound called Roxarsone in it in order to prevent certain parasitic infections. Maybe it is still used, and therefore, so was the chicken. Soil fumigants and fertilizers may contain arsenic, and therefore, so might fruits and vegetables grown in that soil. Crops and well water drawn from deep wells on such land may often contain arsenic. Second-hand tobacco smoke also contains substantial quantities of arsenic.

CARDIOVASCULAR CONSEQUENCES

First of all, we know that it forms a direct complex with glutathione, so having enough glutathione around is a positive thing to remove arsenic via the urine. However, it also means it *depletes your glutathione* stores. We are still trying to investigate directly what happens to the heart as a direct result of arsenic exposure. We know that, like all metal ions, it causes the generation of reactive oxygen species (ROS), which causes the increased formation of oxidized LDL (ox-LDL), which may increase the atherogenic process.

CADMIUM

Cadmium is a highly toxic metal that you might not be as familiar with, but it is ubiquitous, not easily excreted, and highly persistent. Cigarette smoke is a big source of cadmium exposure,[53] and this occurs because the tobacco plant is very efficient at absorbing and concentrating cadmium from the soil and accumulating it

---

53. Nordberg GF, Nogawa K, Nordberg M, Friberg LT. In: Cadmium. Third Edition. Nordberg GF, Fowler BA, Nordberg M, Friberg LT, editors. Elsevier: Handbook on the Toxicology of Metals; 2007. pp. 445–486

in the leaf.[54] You might remember the nickel-cadmium batteries that were all over the place. Tires and rubber products were often made with cadmium, as were pigments for paint. Cadmium yellow, cadmium red, and cadmium orange were actual paint colors (usually as oil paints). Cadmium is bound to proteins, and is not easily excreted, so its half-life can be extremely long: up to 19 years in the liver and up to 38 years in the kidney.[55] Looking at a variety of studies, the cardiovascular risk due to cadmium exposure appears to be approximately up to a factor of 1.5 times greater (death due to CVD).[56] Not extreme, but consistent. Moreover, cadmium also depletes glutathione, and has demonstrated its own independent risk factors for atherosclerosis, including increased IMT (intima-media thickness) and carotid artery plaque.[57]

COBALT

Cobalt, although a rare source of exposure, is used in hip replacements as cobalt-chromium alloys. They have been shown to leach out of the alloy and become cardiotoxic. I should state emphatically that these are *inorganic* cobalt salts, *not methylcobalamin or cyanocobalamin*, which are Vitamin B-12. Those are *organic* forms of cobalt and will not hurt you.

EDTA TREATMENTS: MY VIEW

The TACT trial turned the cardiology world upside down. While

54. Wagner GJ, Yeargan R. Variation in cadmium accumulation potential and tissue distribution of cadmium in tobacco. Plant physiology. 1986;82(1):274–279.
55. Jarup L, Berglund M, Elinder CG, Nordberg G, Vahter M. Health effects of cadmium exposure--a review of the literature and a risk estimate. Scandinavian journal of work, environment & health. 1998;(24 Suppl 1):1–51
56. Tellez-Plaza M, Jones MR, Dominguez-Lucas A, Guallar E, Navas-Acien A. Cadmium exposure and clinical cardiovascular disease: a systematic review. Current atherosclerosis reports. 2013;15(10):356.
57. Messner B, Knoflach M, Seubert A, et al. Cadmium is a novel and independent risk factor for early atherosclerosis mechanisms and in vivo relevance. Arterioscler Thromb Vasc Biol. 2009;29:1392–1398.

we are waiting for TACT2 to reconfirm the initial results, I am offering the TACT protocol to my patients with some special improvements/modification on that protocol, using the knowledge I have just discussed with you.

As demonstrated by these examples and citations, all of these dangerous heavy metals generate reactive oxygen species and deplete your glutathione stores. Therefore, I add a glutathione treatment (separately, of course). That way, we allow the disodium EDTA to chelate out two major classes of compounds: (1) **the calcium** (which is the **plaque** clogging your arteries); and (2) **the heavy metals**.

Then, we replenish your body with a **glutathione treatment** to restore what you've lost. All of this is done under my medical direction and supervision, and you will still take whatever your normal medical treatment is, should you still need it. This is not a substitute for other medical treatment. All of this will be part and parcel of my B-100 plan, and we will be very excited to see what results we can generate with our patient population!

CHAPTER 8

MACRO- AND MICRONUTRIENT DEFICIENCY

It should be little surprise to you by now that the nutrients we take in as part of our diets should have an effect on our hearts. We have talked about how the fifty-plus-year "fad" of low-fat diets, promoted by the American Heart Association (AHA) as "heart-healthy," tended to make matters worse. These low-fat substitutes were actually artificial *trans* fats that had been manufactured, which cause inflammation and raise the risk of heart disease. They also added considerably more sugar, or worse—high-fructose corn syrup—to improve the taste of these "low-fat" products, which had lost considerable flavor by the reduction in fat. Because, as TV Chef Paula Deen has correctly pointed out in her inimitable Southern drawl, "Fat is flavor, y'all!" And, even if the manufacturer does not add sugar, you as consumer do, by eating it from other sources.

It is human nature that your brain and taste buds will find something else to eat to compensate for what you feel is lacking, and, unfortunately for humans, sugar will usually fill the bill— **especially if we are deficient in other macro- and micro-nutrients!** Therefore, it is critical to examine what these nutrients are, and what their deficiencies mean in terms of heart disease.

WHAT ARE MACRONUTRIENTS AND MICRONUTRIENTS? WHAT'S THE DIFFERENCE?

Macronutrients

Traditionally, **macronutrients** are considered to be the nutrients your body requires in large amounts for its essential nutrition. These have normally been defined to include proteins (made up of amino acids), fats (including polyunsaturated, monounsaturated, or saturated fatty acids), and carbohydrates (including starches and sugars). Interestingly, one research paper[58] includes "[c]alcium, as well as magnesium, sodium, and potassium" as "examples of macronutrients, and as such, are crucial for homeostasis." As we will see, while this may have been a rather avant-garde position in 2007, it was a prescient position given what we now know.

Micronutrients

Conversely, compared to macronutrients, **micronutrients** are required in small amounts. Most people think of them as "vitamins and minerals." Some people have defined micronutrients as being required in "trace amounts," but I think this is misleading, because it can confuse people with the term "trace minerals," which are indeed only required in extremely small quantities. Micronutrients include pretty much all the vitamins you have heard of, including the water-soluble vitamins (B-complex vitamins and Vitamin C) and the fat-soluble vitamins (Vitamins A, D, E, and K); as well as what are sometimes called the *macrominerals* because they are present in the largest quantities in your body—**calcium, magnesium, potassium, sodium,** and **phosphorus**—and the *trace minerals*, or *microminerals*, which are present in very small quantities, which I'll bet you probably never even knew were in your body at all: metals like copper, chromium (no, not the toxic chromium (VI) discussed in the movie *Erin Brockovich*, but the type of chromium that's in your

---

58. Newman KP, Bhattacharya SK, Munir A, Davis RC, Soberman JE, Ramanathan KB. Macro- and micronutrients in patients with congestive heart failure, particularly African-Americans. Vasc. Health and Risk Manag. 2007;3(5):743-747.

body that is natural, and regulates your body's glucose levels), molybdenum, manganese, selenium and cobalt.

"Wait a minute, Dr. B," you might be thinking. "Didn't you just tell us cobalt was a toxic heavy metal, in the very last chapter?" Yes, I did. But if you were paying close attention, I also reminded you that an atom of cobalt, when at the center of Vitamin B-12, a.k.a. cyanocobalamin, or its methylated form, methylcobalamin, was harmless, because it was organic, not inorganic or metallic cobalt. It turns out that cobalt, in the organic form, which is obtained through food, not only helps us biosynthesize Vitamin B-12 (accomplished by bacteria in our gut microbiome), but also plays a significant role in the formation of amino acids, certain proteins in nerve cells, and even in the synthesis of neurotransmitters, all of which are crucial for us to be able to function normally.[59]

MACRONUTRIENT DEFICIENCIES AND HEART DISEASE

Let's first take macronutrients as they are defined: Proteins, carbohydrates, and fats. I don't think that too many of us reading this book are *deficient* in carbohydrates or fats. That would be very hard to do in today's America. I suppose it is possible that if you have been excluding *proteins* and been eating nothing but carbs, you could be protein-deficient, or you could also be protein-deficient via what is called small intestinal bacterial overgrowth (back to that gut microbiome again!). If you have an imbalance of the wrong kind of bacteria growing in your small intestine, you may well be *eating* enough protein, but these bacteria are interfering with your body's ability to digest and absorb it into usable calories. Once again, an inflammatory process, such as inflammatory bowel disease (IBD), or Crohn's disease, or a protein-losing enteropathy, could be causing the problem.

---

59. Czarnek K, Terpiłowska S, Siwicki AK. Selected aspects of the action of cobalt ions in the human body. Cent Eur J Immunol. 2015;40(2):236-242.

These may not be obvious things to the general practitioner, and sometimes, a series of blood, breath, and stool tests may be required to find out what is really going on in such a patient.[60]

MACRONUTRIENTS (DEFINED AS MACROMINERALS)

For the purposes of the rest of this chapter, let's define the macronutrients like the paper I mentioned earlier did: "Calcium, as well as magnesium, sodium, and potassium." In other words, the macrominerals, as we defined them earlier, other than phosphorus. The reason for this is that these macrominerals are mega-important to your heart health, and we are in the midst of a major deficiency of at least a couple of them. Especially magnesium. But let's concentrate on the first two to start.

CALCIUM DEFICIENCY

When you think of calcium, you probably think of your mother telling you to drink your milk, or TV commercials telling you to drink milk, or take calcium supplements, because they build strong bones and healthy teeth. Well, that's true. In fact, some 99% of your body's calcium is found in your teeth and bones. But did you know that calcium serves other important functions too? Functions like controlling muscle contractility—including the heart (it's a muscle)—transmission of nerve impulses, and—quite significantly where we are concerned—contraction and relaxation of vascular smooth muscle, namely, the type of muscle that makes up the vascular endothelium (blood vessel walls). So, for example, too little calcium in your blood just might result in your heart muscle not having as great of a contractile force as it should (the technical term is *inotropy*, and a drug like digitalis is referred to as giving a "positive inotropic effect" because it increases the contractile force of your heart muscle). Now,

---

60. Karp, SM, Koch, T.R., Mechanisms of Macronutrient Deficiency and Associated Clinical Conditions. Dis Mon. 2006;52:164-169.

certainly, we have known that this is true of patients in heart failure, for example.

Intracellularly (inside the heart muscle cell), there are calcium channels that create action potentials. This process is very tightly controlled; loss of this control causes an overload of intracellular calcium, and arrhythmia, which in turn can cause sudden cardiac death. This control is lost with most of the cardiomyopathies and congestive heart failure. This is why some patients take "calcium channel blockers," such as verapamil, which prevent the uncoordinated, willy-nilly firing of those channels, and thus stop arrhythmias in that fashion.

Extracellularly, i.e., *outside* the heart muscle cell, such as in the bloodstream, then, it is low levels of calcium that seem to cause the problem: just the reverse of what we described in the paragraph above. The delicate balance of extracellular calcium levels is a constant dance between how much calcium you take in through what you eat; how much is actually absorbed through your intestines; how much is excreted through your kidneys; (and a lot of people forget this one, but that's why we all worry about calcium, right?) how much is turned over through bone remodeling. And that process is controlled by two main hormones: One of them, you probably know, Vitamin D3. Yes, boys and girls! Vitamin D is a hormone—even though it's also all-natural and comes from the sun. (Free-range, no antibiotics, and fair trade, too! And, did I mention, Vitamin D is also 100% gluten-free?)

The other hormone that you probably are not as familiar with is parathyroid hormone (PTH, for short). PTH has nothing to do with your thyroid: it's produced by the four parathyroid glands, tiny glands that look no bigger than grains of rice that sit nestled just under your thyroid gland. Barely visible, the powerful parathyroid and their PTH they produce pack one heck of a punch, exerting tyrannical control, in tandem with Vitamin D, over calcium levels throughout your body. If PTH levels go haywire, watch out—calcium levels go crazy. The result? Well, paresthesias, which we talked about before (the needles and pins). And then, there's tetany. That means muscle cramps that stay cramped. Muscles that just freeze, Botox-style, but when you didn't go looking for that Botox effect. Lockjaw is a good example of this. If it hits the diaphragm muscles, or the intercostal muscles (between the ribs), guess what, you can't breathe! No bueno! So, low PTH, low calcium, is generally how it goes.

We know that in patients who have clinical syndromes where they are *hypocalcemic*, i.e., where they are dangerously low in calcium, they will be at risk for life-threatening cardiovascular events.[61] But, according to a recent study[62] published by researchers at the venerable Cedars-Sinai Heart Institute, it turns out that a lot more people who may have had what were considered to be "low-normal"—and certainly not "deficient"—levels of calcium may be at heightened risk for heart disease. This study compared cases of sudden cardiac arrest (SCA) with matched controls from another large, population-based study. So, by matched controls, we mean that they also had a generally "matching" diagnosis – in this study, coronary artery disease (CAD), as opposed to a healthy control group.

The data revealed that, in blood drawn within 90 days of the sudden cardiac arrest, blood calcium levels lower than 8.95 mg/dL were associated with a 2.3-fold increase in odds of having an SCA as compared with levels higher than 9.55 mg/dL. And for every 1-unit change, they had a 1.6-fold increase. Now what is interesting to note here is that 8.95 mg/dL is *not* a very low number for serum calcium. In fact, although the FDA "normal range" is 9-11 mg/dL, some labs have their "low" cut point as low as 8.6 mg/dL. Although this study is not without its flaws—I

---

61. Cecchi E, Grossi F, Rossi M, et al., Severe hypocalcemia and life-threatening ventricular arrhythmias: case report and proposal of a diagnostic and therapeutic algorithm. Clin Cases Miner Bone Metab. 2015 Sep-Dec;12(3):265-8.
62. Lee, H-C. Serum Calcium: A Sudden Cardiac Arrest Risk Factor. Mayo Clinic Proceedings, Volume 92, Issue 10, 1466 – 1468.

wish it had been done using *ionized calcium*, which is a much more reliable measurement—it has certainly added to the debate because it states that "low-normal" blood calcium is an *independent risk factor* (meaning that they said, have corrected for other confounding factors that might have affected the data) for sudden cardiac arrhythmia.

But Dr. B., Wasn't There a Study Saying Calcium Caused Coronary Artery Disease and Heart Attacks?

You may have remembered a few years ago when everyone was panicking about taking too many calcium supplements because they thought coronary artery calcification might be the result. I wrote about it in our newsletter and blog. This is because there were a few preliminary studies —especially the MESA study— that appeared to be alarming in this regard but were certainly not conclusive. And whereas in 2013, it may have *appeared* that there was a 1:1 correlation between our taking even modest amounts of calcium supplements and them being inevitably and irretrievably deposited on the walls of our arteries and rendering them into human White Cliffs of Dover[63] through which blood may occasionally hope to pass, since then, other studies have come out showing that slightly higher levels of calcium do not pose any cardiac risk. Only if the calcium levels are kept very high and for a long time does CV disease seem to develop in response.

In my opinion, these results tell me we really need to re-evaluate what the lower boundary of "normal" calcium is: Perhaps it may be closer to 8.8-8.9 mg/dL than 8.6, and perhaps we may need to treat to at least 9.0; however, it remains to be seen if these results can be replicated. But for now, especially if needed to forestall osteoporosis, for example, or even, let's say, hypothetically at this point, to prevent SCA, I would not be averse to patients having a reasonable amount of calcium, but dietary sources are always preferred to supplements. So, at this point, like I am

---

63. The famous White Cliffs of Dover, in Dover, England, are composed mainly of limestone, or calcium carbonate.

fond of reminding my patients, with so much of our bodies, but particularly the heart, with calcium, you have to be Goldilocks, and say: "Not too little, not too much—just right!"

MAGNESIUM DEFICIENCY

Magnesium is a mineral that can have major effects on the heart: it serves as a "counterbalance" of sorts to calcium. Too much magnesium or too little magnesium—either condition can cause arrhythmias that can result in sudden cardiac death. But it is also one of the most *vital* minerals to your heart, and one in which Americans are woefully deficient. Quite the paradox, n'est-ce pas? I thought so, too. In 2009, no less august a body than the World Health Organization published a report[64] suggesting that over 75% of Americans are seriously deficient in magnesium.

There is a growing body of evidence that suggests that low serum magnesium levels increase your risk of death from coronary heart disease or sudden cardiac death.[65] In the Atherosclerosis Risk in Communities (ARIC) Study,[66] the study participants in the highest quartile of serum magnesium levels were 40% less likely to suffer sudden cardiac death (SCD) than those in the lowest quartile, showing that low magnesium levels are an independent risk factor for sudden cardiac death. Further, a recent Chinese study found that increased dietary magnesium intake is associated with a reduced risk of stroke, heart failure, diabetes, and all-cause mortality (although it showed no effect on total CVD).[67]

64. World Health Organization. Calcium and Magnesium in Drinking Water: Public Health Significance. Geneva: World Health Organization Press; 2009.
65. Kieboom BC, Niemeijer MN, Leening MJ, et al. Serum magnesium and the risk of death from coronary heart disease and sudden cardiac death. J Am Heart Assoc. 2016;5.
66. Peacock, J. M., T. Ohira, et al. (2010). "Serum magnesium and risk of sudden cardiac death in the Atherosclerosis Risk in Communities (ARIC) Study." Am Heart J 160(3): 464-70.
67. Fang, X, Wang, K, Han, D. Dietary magnesium intake and the risk of cardiovascular disease, type 2 diabetes, and all-cause mortality: a dose–response meta-analysis of prospective cohort studies. BMC Medicine 2016. 14:210.

What is amazing to me is that George Lundberg, M.D., who for over 20 years was the Editor-in-Chief of *JAMA* (*Journal of the American Medical Association*), and then went on to run Medscape (website) as Editor, and continues there as Editor-at-Large today, is extolling the benefits of magnesium supplements, and warning his fellow doctors about the dangers of magnesium deficiency. This man is not exactly some hippie Alternative Medicine doctor. Dr. Lundberg is a mainstream pillar of establishment medicine, yet he is ahead of the curve on magnesium. He knows that most of this country is terribly deficient. He points out that foods high in magnesium include: dark leafy greens like kale (trendy right now!), chard, and spinach; tree nuts and peanuts; seeds; oily fish, such as salmon; beans, lentils, legumes, and whole grains; avocado, yogurt, bananas, dried fruit; and, what I'm sure will be a very easy thing for many of you to incorporate into your diets—dark chocolate (yes, it's high in magnesium!).

Dr. Lundberg states that he takes 400 mg. of magnesium as the citrate salt. And that's a good, sensible start. It's available commercially as magnesium oxide, chloride, and also as glycinate and as organic "chelated" forms. Now, the thing is, you can't really take too much orally: it will just upset your stomach: That's why many laxatives are also made of magnesium citrate. (Milk of Magnesia, anyone?) But, if you really want to get better absorption, and balance out the magnesium and calcium ratios (usually 1:2), but I can help you because this should be adjusted along with your medications, IV therapy is really the way to go. That way, you bypass the intestinal tract completely—no upset stomach. That's what a lot of my patients love about it. But whatever you choose, make sure to take a good quality Vitamin D3 along with your calcium and magnesium.

The other macrominerals are potassium and sodium. Do not try to mess with these on your own. As a doctor, I will give out potassium supplements if you are low in potassium, or at risk for becoming low in potassium, such as if you are on a diuretic, but otherwise, this is not a do-it-yourself proposition. Leave it to the pros.

CHAPTER 9

GENETICS

"Biology is destiny." This quote, often incorrectly attributed to Sigmund Freud, circa 1924, would sometimes seem even more true in today's era, where we have sequenced the entire human genome (in 2003), routinely screen for genetic diseases, and have developed many medications using genetic engineering techniques. However, it is very simplistic, and often does not tell the whole story. Often, it is completely wrong, and is *not* destiny, because environmental factors override someone's biology (genetics). Many times, a combination of both genetic risk factors and environmental influences is at play when considering a "multifactorial" disease, such as cardiovascular disease or cancer.

THE DIATHESIS-STRESS MODEL

The world of clinical psychology actually put forth this model, but I have always liked it, because it describes many diseases accurately. You must first have a genetic predisposition (what they call here the *diathesis*), but only when that predisposition is "activated" or "triggered" by various types of *stress* in the environment—which could be very broadly defined—does the full-blown disease or condition manifest itself. Visualize, for example, a person with a genetic predisposition to skin cancer. (There are various genetic syndromes, such as ataxia-telangiectasia syndrome, which makes one especially at risk, but also, just being albino, or even being a redhead with very fair skin and blue eyes, especially if they have a lot of freckles!) But that's just the *predisposition.*

In order to actually develop *skin cancer,* that person needs to be exposed to UV radiation from the sun (or a tanning bed), which directly damages their DNA. Exposing the skin to chemical carcinogens would also cause the same result. However, you can easily see how this "one-two punch" mechanism results in cancer. This is probably a very reasonable explanation for many kinds of diseases, because it takes into account the interaction between someone's genetic predisposition, that is, their innate, built-in vulnerability, and Mother Nature's multitudinous environmental insults and assaults, which run the gamut from chemical and radiological to bacterial, viral, helminthic, rickettsial, and even prionic.

A LITTLE BASIC GENETICS REFRESHER COURSE

If we're going to talk about genetics and heart disease, a crash refresher course in genetics is in order. Now, as you all probably remember, there would be no such thing as modern genetics if it weren't for an Austrian monk—Gregor Mendel—who got so bored with the whole "monk" thing day after day that he decided to break up the monastic monotony by doing some experiments involving selective breeding of pea plants. (Hey, for *him,* that was exciting, and a good thing it was, too!) Actually, Mendel *originally* wanted to do his selective breeding studies on mice, but the story goes that, at the time, his bishop felt very strongly that any experiments that would require Mendel to watch animals have sex would be very inappropriate and unseemly, and immediately vetoed the idea. So, pea plants it was!

Greg carefully crossed purebred varieties of plants, and then observed the variation in the next generation (the hybrids). The results were unexpected: A purple-flowered *purebred* pea plant crossed with a white-flowered *purebred* pea plant yielded *only* purple-flowered progeny. How could that be? But then, when he self-fertilized those purple hybrids, the next generation was mainly purple, but not completely: There was a distinct 3:1 ratio of purple: white-flowered pea plants. This result led Mendel to develop the theory of dominance and recessive inheritance, which describes why the first cross only resulted in purple flowers. This is because the "purple" trait (the gene for purple) is "dominant" over the gene for the gene for "white." The diagram below explains this concept nicely:

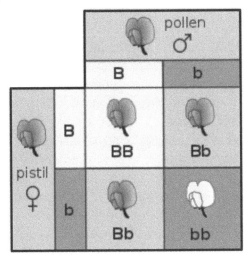

Diagram 1 - Self-Fertilization cross.
(Details in box below)

A Punnett square showing a self-fertilization cross like that performed by Gregor Mendel of the F1. Diagram courtesy of Madeleine Price Ball, Creative Commons License.

In the above diagram, the letter B represents the "purple" *allele*, or variety of the flower-color gene, while the lowercase "b" represents the "white" allele. It takes two alleles, one from each parent, to make up your genotype. A gene is actually located at a specific place (called a locus) on one of your (or, in this case, the pea plant's) chromosomes.

We now know that, in a cross of two purple *hybrids*, 1 out of 4 will be the genotype BB and will be purple, 2 out of 4 will be the genotype Bb—and will likewise be purple—and finally, the remaining 1 out of 4 will be the genotype bb, and will be white. Because 3 out of 4 are purple, purple is dominant over white, and this is also why the white is represented as the lowercase "b," rather than the capital "B." Note that it only takes one capital B to make a flower purple, and it will be purple even though there is a lowercase "b" there, because "B" is dominant over "b." Likewise, for the same reason, you need two lowercase "b" alleles to have a white flower because "b" is recessive.

If you have two alleles of the same type (both "capital," or both "lowercase," one from each parent), that is called *homozygous* (homozygous dominant or homozygous recessive, respectively). If you have one allele of each, dominant and recessive, that is known as *heterozygous*. This is important when looking at inheritance patterns of genetic diseases. Further, inheritance can be described as autosomal (genes on the 22 pairs of non-sex chromosomes) or sex-linked (genes on the X or Y chromosomes). Genetic diseases with an autosomal-dominant mode of inheritance— Huntington's disease is a classic example— can hit not only patients, but their families— particularly hard. For example, if a patient with Huntington's disease who does not know she has the condition—which is, unfortunately, a common situation because it may not manifest symptoms until after age 40-45—marries a man who has not been tested, there is already a 50% probability that she will pass her Huntington's allele onto her child with the man, regardless of what his genetic testing reveals. If he is a carrier, he will have a 50% chance of passing on *his* Huntington's gene. And because it is dominant, it only takes *one* copy of the mutant allele to cause the disease, which is ultimately debilitating and fatal.

For people who may be at risk for Huntington's but who have decided not to have children, the fact that no cure is yet available, and the devastating outcome implied by a positive test result has caused a sizable proportion of such people to elect *not* to get genetic testing. Also, people in that situation have worried about being discriminated against for having a terminal illness. Those can be some really serious and valid concerns.

Thankfully, the strides that genetic testing has made in areas like cancer screening. (Just as an example, testing for the BRCA-1 gene has enabled many women to become aware of their elevated breast-cancer risk, and take preventive action, including prophylactic mastectomies, that has saved countless lives.) I am here to tell you now that today, with the current state of knowledge in my practice, in terms of preventing heart disease, in terms of substantially reducing your risk of getting a heart attack, knowing your genetic risk factors can be a powerful advantage.

AHA AND JACC GUIDELINES ONLY COVER "MOST PEOPLE" IN AVERAGE SITUATIONS

That isn't Customized to Your Personal Situation, and That's Not Acceptable When Your Life Is at Stake!

Sometimes the Guidelines Result in Unnecessary Prescriptions that Patients Can't Tolerate:

Maria G., one of the patients in my practice is in her late 70s. For 20 years, Maria had stubbornly-elevated cholesterol levels. Per the AHA guidelines, I put her on several high-dose statins. But her cholesterol stayed high, no matter what I did. And she had bad side-effects from the statins. They were upsetting her quality of life, which had otherwise been good. Otherwise, she seemed healthy. I noticed that high cholesterol ran in her family. So, on a hunch, I ran a coronary artery calcium (CAC) CT scan. I wanted to see how badly her coronary arteries were calcified to assess her heart attack risk directly. To my absolute shock, she had a CAC score of *zero*. There were no calcium deposits on her arterial walls. So, that told me that, in her case, I could safely take her off statin therapy, as the side effects were not worth it, and that her "high cholesterol" had caused her absolutely no coronary artery disease. Would I do this with all of my patients who complained about their statins? Of course not. But my point is, every patient is an individual.

THE STANDARD GUIDELINES DON'T CATCH PEOPLE AT RISK FOR A HEART ATTACK

On the other side of the coin, I remember another patient of mine, (Jay V), from a few years ago, a high-powered executive who came to see me between business meetings. He exercised regularly two to three times a week. He was the proverbial "picture of health." He was not overweight, did not smoke, and his labs were perfect in every way. A month before he came to see me to establish cardiac care, he suffered a massive heart attack that began with a clot in the left anterior descending artery—this is known as a "widow-maker" heart attack, and, as the name implies, is almost universally fatal. He, fortunately, survived. As we later discovered, the standard blood work did not uncover important genetic risk factors that predisposed him to this type of serious heart attack.

So, unlike other kinds of genetic testing, where I can understand people's reticence to be hit with horrible news and not be able to do anything about it, today, the types of tests that I use in my practice provide you, the patient, with actionable knowledge, because once you can identify what a positive test result means, you can take specific medical, and perhaps even surgical interventions (if necessary) in order to change your odds and make them in your favor. That's the difference. Let me give you some examples (see below) of what we are doing now, in our practice, and how your genetics can work to your advantage, by using diagnostic tests as an early warning system:

CLOT OR NOT?

When it gets right down to it, a number of our genetic tests revolve around genes that affect clotting factors, because if those genes are mutated from their normal state, your blood will be more likely to form clots. This is not a good thing, because, as we all know by now, the formation of a clot is a prelude to a heart attack. The increased tendency of blood to form clots is called *hypercoagulability.*

GENETIC TESTS FOR HYPERCOAGULABILITY

1. Prothrombin Mutation

One of the standard tests we do on patients is their PTT, (partial thromboplastin time) or prothrombin time (PT). If your PTT, or PT is down, your blood is clotting too fast, and that is not normal! If you have a mutation in the prothrombin gene, your body makes too much of the prothrombin protein, which your body uses to help blood clot. This makes you much more susceptible to DVTs (deep venous thromboses) as well as heart attacks. Therefore, it is important to test for the genetic mutation itself.

If we find you are positive for it, we can take action by giving you anticoagulant therapy and monitoring you closely, so you are much less likely to have a clot, and thus, a heart attack.

2. Factor V Leiden

Factor V Leiden is another genetic mutation that is not usually screened for. Factor V (the normal gene) is a blood-clotting factor. However, Factor V Leiden is the mutant form of the gene. It is inherited as an autosomal dominant, making 50% of offspring affected. It results in a hypercoagulable state, which, in turn, causes the blood to be more likely to clot, and therefore, increases heart attack risk. Factor V Leiden is an important part of the preventive program in my practice.

As with prothrombin mutations, a positive test result for this mutation can sometimes be addressed with anticoagulant treatment.

Lipoprotein(a) and Heart Attack Risk: Taking the Lead in Diagnosis

When you think "lipoprotein," you think "LDL" or "HDL." That's natural. But there are other lipoproteins that you, and more importantly, the medical community, should be aware of. And Lipoprotein(a) – Lp(a) – is a pretty important one. What many people, and indeed, many other doctors, still do not realize, is that elevated levels of Lipoprotein(a) can cause a significantly increased risk of cardiovascular disease, and nearly 20% of the population of the United States have those elevated levels!

LP(A) IS PERSONAL TO ME

You see, Lipoprotein (a), a.k.a. Lp(a), is actually an area of very special interest to me. My mother-in-law (before I got married) died because of a heart attack due to chronically elevated Lp(a) levels. Her brother, who was only in his late forties, had multiple PTCAs (percutaneous transluminal coronary angioplasties) because of repeated coronary artery blockages due to the problem, and my brother-in-law's numbers are sky high! Many cardiologists don't know the extent of the problem and worse, don't know how to treat it.

Lipoprotein(a) = An LDL-like Particle Linked to apo(a) Protein

Lipoprotein(a) is a weird kind of lipoprotein: One part is an LDL-like particle. As such, that part of the molecule will readily penetrate the vascular endothelium, where it can undergo oxidation to the oxidized form (Ox-LDL). This step is necessary to pave the way for an atherosclerotic plaque to form. Thus, the LDL-like half of the molecule is considered to be *proatherogenic*, or promoting atherosclerosis. That much is straightforward. But how about the other part of the molecule, the long, covalently linked apo(a) protein? Well, as it turns out, this bad boy is a 2-for-1 special: The other half of the molecule—the apo(a) protein—shares a structural homology with (meaning the protein is evolutionarily very similar to) plasminogen.[68] What's plasminogen? Well, if you remember tissue plasminogen activator (tPA), that was the big clot-busting wonder drug of a decade or two ago. Larry King's cardiologist gave it to him and saved his life. Without getting into the mechanism of how it works, it is thought that the apolipoprotein(a) part of the molecule is pro-thrombogenic[69] (promotes blood clots), so the net effect of the two parts of Lp(a) is truly the worst of both worlds.[70] The two things in combination (clot plus arterial blockage), logically, will drastically increase the chance of not only heart attack (which proceeds via atherosclerotic and thrombotic mechanisms), but also pure thrombotic events, such as DVTs, as well as other events such as peripheral artery disease and stroke.

This Lp(a) sounds horrible! Therefore, shouldn't we eliminate this horrible mutant gene?

First of all, Lp(a) is *not* a mutation. Secondly, everybody makes lipoprotein(a), so we can't get rid of it. (As it turns out, there probably was some evolutionary purpose for it—having to do

---

68. Boffa MB, Marcovina SM, Koschinsky ML. Lipoprotein(a) as a risk factor for atherosclerosis and thrombosis: mechanistic insights from animal models. Clin Biochem. 2004 May;37(5):333-43.

69. Hansen PR. [Lipoprotein(a): a link between thrombosis and atherosclerosis?] [Article in Danish] Ugeskr. Laeger. 1993 May 17;155(20):1527-30.

70. This study says it beautifully: "Lipoprotein (a) has both atherogenic and prothrombotic properties. The atherogenic potential is mainly due to the presence of the LDL particle, which promotes atherosclerosis via Lp(a)-derived cholesterol entrapment in the intima, via inflammatory cell recruitment, via the binding of proinflammatory-oxidized phospholipids, and by adversely affecting endothelium-dependent arterial reactivity. The thrombogenic potential is exerted mainly via apolipoprotein(a), which has structural homology with plasminogen and inhibits fibrinolysis by blocking plasmin generation on fibrin."

with wound healing—which is why there is a clotting function associated with it.) It is the *excess* production of Lp(a) that is an inherited trait, however, and which is clinically proven to cause real problems: coronary heart disease, atherosclerosis, stroke, and calcified aortic stenosis. Remember I've talked to you about your heart valves and your arteries getting calcium deposits? (Like the CAC score I was discussing to measure calcium in coronary arteries?) Well, as it turns out, Lp(a) promotes this process, and it's frighteningly effective at doing so.

20% OF AMERICANS HAVE ELEVATED LP(A) LEVELS, PUTTING THEM AT VERY HIGH RISK FOR CARDIOVASCULAR DISEASE

The point is, 20% of us have *elevated levels* of Lp(a)—defined as >50 mg/dL[71] (the normal range is considered <30 mg/dL). Clinically, an elevated Lp(a) level (>50 mg/dL) was correlated with a nearly three-fold increased risk of acute coronary syndrome in young and middle-aged patients. Patients who would never think of themselves as being at risk for heart disease. In other words, this is scary stuff! Unfortunately, many physicians think that, simply because Lp(a) is a lipoprotein, statins will work to lower its blood levels. Not so. Paradoxically, statins will *raise* your Lp(a) level. This makes it even more of a challenge to treat. Quite a few of my patients who have come to see me after seeing other providers were quite surprised to hear *that* bit of news. And, although it isn't *easy* to bring those levels down, we are working on possible solutions to that problem and I am excited to announce that as of the writing of this book, one treatment protocol has shown significantly lower Lp(a) levels. FDA is currently investigating this form of therapy for general use.

---

71. Rallidis, Loukianos S. et al. High levels of lipoprotein (a) and premature acute coronary syndrome. Atherosclerosis, Volume 269, 29 – 34.

APOE GENOTYPE TESTING

APOE is a gene which codes for the protein ApoE, or Apolipoprotein E. Yes, I know what you're thinking. Another lipoprotein, Bereliani? But trust me, this lipoprotein is *really interesting.* There are polymorphisms, or variations in several of the alleles on this gene which are significant, known as E2, E3, and E4. Remember, a person has two copies of each gene, so their genotype might look like [E2, E2], or [E2, E3], or [E3, E3]. Or [E3, E4], or [E4, E4]. You get the picture. If you have the E2 allele, either one or two copies of it, it is protective against cardiovascular disease, while the E4 allele seems to increase cardiovascular disease risk, according to several studies, which have been fairly consistent over the years.[72, 73]

But, as the late-night infomercials say, "But wait! There's more! Because if you act now and order your APOE genotype test, you'll see that you don't just get a test for heart disease. *No, sir! You'll get to see what happens when you and your loved ones get to be **old-timers**! Does your APOE genotype put you at high risk for **Alzheimer's**? Let us help.*"

With apologies for the cornball copy, it is in fact true that one of the surprising things that a number of my patients have discovered is that the APOE genotypes have had a long-standing association with other conditions besides cardiovascular, and that one of the most significant of these to me has been the connection to Alzheimer's disease. It appears that, much like in cardiovascular disease, the E4 allele was the really bad one, and patients who had either one or both E4 alleles seemed to be much more likely to be later diagnosed with Alzheimer's disease. In fact, in one study, subjects with one copy of the E4 allele (genotype [E3,E4])

72. Bennet AM, Di Angelantonio E, Ye Z. Association of apolipoprotein E genotypes with lipid levels and coronary risk. JAMA. 2007 Sep 19;298(11):1300-11.
73. Zhang Y, Tang H-Q, Peng W-J, Zhang B-B, Liu M. Meta-analysis for the Association of Apolipoprotein E ε2/ε3/ε4 Polymorphism with Coronary Heart Disease. Chinese Medical Journal. 2015;128(10):1391-1398.

had a 21% (male carriers) to 30% (female carriers) lifetime risk of developing Alzheimer's disease, whereas those with the homozygous genotype [E4,E4] had a 51%(male carriers) to 60% (for female carriers) lifetime risk of developing Alzheimer's disease.[74] Clearly, these sorts of results militate for genetic testing and counseling. Especially if there are specific medication and lifestyle interventions that can be undertaken in order to change these grim figures.

OTHER IMPORTANT GENETIC TESTS

<u>MTHFR and Homocysteine:</u>

Although not terribly well known, elevated levels of the amino acid homocysteine have long been recognized as a risk factor for heart attack. One problem is that testing for homocysteine is not commonly employed. However, it is usually a fairly reliable indicator that your lipid panel may also be off. And it is usually a marker that shows up in association with inflammation. But what happens with a positive result? How do you reduce the homocysteine level? And what is the root cause of the high homocysteine level? As to the first question, you can give the patient folic acid (I prefer methylfolate). As to the second question, that is not always easily answered. And for the answer, I may often have to turn to genetic testing for the MTHFR gene. MTHFR stands for MethyleneTetraHydroFolate Reductase, the enzyme that reduces **5,10-**_methylene_tetrahydrofolate (5,10-CH2-THF) to **10-methyl**tetrahydrofolate, which in turn, acts as a cofactor for the conversion of homocysteine, which can build up to toxic levels, back to methionine, which is an essential amino acid.

So if I have given somebody methylfolate supplements, and their homocysteine level has not been going down, and I don't understand, or my patient doesn't understand what might be

---

74. Genin E, Hannequin D, Wallon D. APOE and Alzheimer disease: a major gene with semi-dominant inheritance. Mol Psychiatry. 2011 Sep;16(9):903-7.

causing the elevated homocysteine levels, I remember all the unusual experiences both my patients and I have gone through. Testing for MTHFR mutations is one way to look for possible issues. The bottom line is that there are now many other precision tests that are now available to me thanks to testing methods and levels of analysis and understanding we simply did not have before.

CHAPTER 10

STRESS

Stress: a simple word, but one which has myriad definitions, each of which, in turn, has ample room for interpretation.

"Stress" could mean *oxidative stress*, which is what we have mainly discussed in this book—the oxidation of LDL, for example, which causes the generation of reactive oxygen species (ROS). These ROS are known as free radicals, which attack cells via chain reactions. This sequence of events, which occurs as part of normal lipid metabolism and respiration, is what we mean by oxidative damage. The [usually] long-term exposure of your body's cells to the insults of ROS—which can be generated not only by respiration and metabolism, but also by exogenous (outside) sources, such as toxic chemicals, ionizing radiation (such as UV-B radiation [the type of solar radiation that causes sunburns], X-rays, gamma-rays, or alpha or beta particles, such as those used in radiation therapy for cancer)—which can, at the extreme end of the spectrum, actually cause direct damage to your DNA, and thus, a mutation to one or more of your genes—is what we mean by "oxidative stress." Or, it could mean *physical stress*, as in running a marathon, or power-lifting.

MENTAL STRESS

By and large, what we usually mean when we say the word "stress" is *emotional stress* (also called mental stress or psychological stress). By this, we are referring to the stress brought about by emotionally traumatic or upsetting life events, which are usually of the *acute* (sudden) variety, but also may be *chronic* (ongoing) in nature. This is the type of stress which we will focus on in this chapter. The overarching question is, can mental stress directly cause cardiovascular diseases like heart attacks and strokes? This has long been an area of intense study by many groups of investigators. The broad-strokes answer seems to be a definite, "Yes." We have all heard of examples of people being stressed, in one way or another, to the point of having a heart attack. If someone points a gun at you, for example, the fright alone can induce a heart attack. The stress of a natural disaster, such as an earthquake or a hurricane, may cause deaths to many of its victims even without inflicting a direct hit on them, simply by virtue of the unexpected shock and enormity that something so fearsome poses, arriving quite literally out of the clear blue sky, raining down utter death and destruction in its wake. If you experience the sudden death of a loved one, it is well known that that experience can also cause you to suffer a heart attack as well. [In Appendix B on page 189, I will discuss the mechanisms by which acute stress causes a heart attack.]

In this chapter, however, I will discuss the effect of CHRONIC stress on cardiovascular health, specifically as it relates to heart attack. Chronic stress refers to a persistent unrelenting emotional stress, be it mild or severe, over months or years. These types of stress are usually related to job, finances, chronic health issues, relationship issues, abandonment issues, abuse, loss or simply mental health issues such as generalized chronic anxiety issues. Chronic stress is rapidly becoming a major risk factor for heart disease in the current world we live in. This is due to ever worsening complexities of our lives compared to many decades ago. So how does chronic (let's say mild) stress could lead to a heart attack over a few years?

1. Stress Hormones
From an evolutionary standpoint, stress hormones were

designed to provide the energy and mental sharpness needed to fight an impending threat to our lives. As its name implies, the stress hormones are secreted in response to stress (any type of stress, be it mental or physical). Imagine a stone-age male hunting for food in jungles encountering a lion or a large poisonous snake. He would need every bit of energy as well as a sharp and focused mind to either FIGHT or escape (FLIGHT) – the so-called *fight-or-flight* response. Furthermore, he would need the energy to be in a readily available form so his brain and heart and the other organs can utilize it immediately.

The body derives energy from three sources: (1) Fat, (2) Protein, and (3) Carbohydrates (sugars). Both fat and protein will need to be converted to carbohydrates in order for the brain, heart and other organs to utilize them. In response to stress, the stress hormones release a large amount of glucose (sugars) to the bloodstream and some of these stress hormones (for example insulin) help transfer these sugars to muscles and the other organs to feed the fuel needed to fight the enemy or the threat. This very efficient and helpful evolutionary mechanism helped humans fight off wild animals, escape from natural disasters and win wars in the stone age and the paleolithic period. Unfortunately, these stress hormones cannot distinguish different types of stress, but get secreted in response to any sort of stress. If you are the type who likes to stay up all night and party, or if you are only getting two hours of sleep a night because you are writing a novel, you can expect to have chronically-elevated stress hormones. Ok, what is the downside of these stress hormones and how could they cause heart disease in the long run?

Stress hormones include the hormones: Cortisol, Epinephrine, Norepinephrine, Dopamine, C-Reactive Protein, Insulin and many more. All these hormones have shown to accelerate atherosclerosis (plaque build-up in the coronary arteries), increase inflammation and cause endothelial dysfunction. As we discussed in the previous chapters, endothelial dysfunction also causes plaque buildup, and both endothelial dysfunction and inflammation can lead to plaque rupture and heart attack. These hormones are also well known to worsen almost all the risk factors involved in the development of a heart attack. Cortisol, epinephrine and norepinephrine increase the blood pressure and vasoconstriction of the arteries of the heart and the rest of the body. Cortisol also causes hyperglycemia (elevated sugar levels) which could lead to diabetes, and Cortisol and Insulin cause weight gain. Epinephrine and Norepinephrine as well as dopamine increase the workload on the heart.

Chronic increase in the workload of the heart causes heart FAILURE as well as heart attack. Some of the markers of stress causing endothelial damage and plaque rupture are IL-6 and IL-16 (InterLeukin). Many studies have shown these markers to go up with stress. These markers have also shown to be elevated in patients just prior to a heart attack. This is therefore, one of the many markers I use to reliably assess one's risk of future heart attack as it relates to one's stress.

2. Other mechanisms

Chronic stress leads to a state of constant activation of the sympathetic nervous system. Our nervous system is comprised of two different systems: The first is the Parasympathetic System – which is comprised of a group of nerves which get activated when we relax. For example, when we eat food, this group of nerves gets activated to help digest the food by increasing the movement of our intestines (a process called Peristalsis). Secondly, the Sympathetic Nervous System, on the other hand, gets activated during a *Fight-or-Flight* response.

Therefore, these are the nerves that get activated in response to stress. The group of nerves adversely affect our heart in two ways. First they cause the secretion of all the stress hormones we discussed above. Second, these nerves directly increase the work of the heart as they directly innervated the heart and the arteries of the body. So they cause chronically higher heart rate and blood pressure as well as our respiratory rate. Over time, this increase in the work of the heart can lead to heart attack and heart failure.

You can understand why, then, a major part of my treatment plan involves identifying and managing the source of stress in our patients.

CHAPTER 11

TELOMERES AND HEART DISEASE

WHAT IS A TELOMERE?

Telomeres are repetitive sequences of DNA, occurring at the ends of chromosomes, made up of the DNA bases thymine, adenine, and guanine in the sequence TTAGGG. They are often compared to the plastic "caps" at the ends of shoelaces. A scientist named Leonard Hayflick observed that certain cells have a limit on the number of times they will divide before they will just *stop* dividing. This principle has been termed *replicative senescence.* So, with each replication, the telomeres become progressively shorter until replicative senescence is reached.[75] The enzyme *telomerase*, on the other hand, can reverse this process. The function of telomerase is generally maintaining telomere length (TL). So, activation of telomerase results in telomere elongation; and regulation of telomerase activity can literally save cells from senescence.[76] Yes, boys and girls, "senescence" is just a fancy word for "aging!" And thus, telomeres may just hold a major key to the mysteries of aging.

75. Wong, JM, Collins, K (2003). Telomere maintenance and disease. The Lancet Vol. 362, No.9388, (2003/9/20 2003), pp. 983-988.
76. Zvereva, MI, Shcherbakova, DM, Dontsova, OA (2010). Telomerase: structure, functions, and activity regulation. Biochemistry (Mosc) Vol. 75, No. 13, (Dec 2010), pp. 1563-1583, 1608-3040 (Electronic) 0006-2979 (Linking).

TELOMERE LENGTH AS A BIOMARKER OF CARDIOVASCULAR DISEASE

There have been multiple studies investigating the relationship between telomere length (TL) and mortality in general, as well as correlating TL specifically with various kinds of diseases, but recently, several studies have identified TL as a very good biomarker for cardiovascular aging. Based on a systematic review of twenty-four studies involving 43,725 participants and 8,400 patients with cardiovascular disease (5,566 with coronary heart disease and 2,834 with cerebrovascular disease), shorter leukocyte (white blood cell) telomere length was found to be an independent risk factor for coronary heart disease (excluding traditional risk factors for CHD), with the pooled relative risk for coronary heart disease being 1.54. That means people with shorter telomeres were 1.54 times as likely to have heart attacks as those with longer telomeres! No statistically relevant association was seen with cerebrovascular disease.

Well, so what, you might be saying? Those telomeres were in *leukocytes*. Well, a study at University of Pennsylvania has shown that this holds true in heart muscle cells (called cardiomyocytes) as well: Shortening of *those* telomeres was directly proven to be associated with heart failure and certain kinds of cardiomyopathy.[77]

SO WHAT CAN WE DO WITH THIS INFORMATION?

We can now test for telomere length. But what if your telomeres are too short? What can we do about it? Well, one thing that we know, and have known for years, is that oxidative stress causes telomere shortening.[78] Therefore, by that logic, reducing

---

77. Sharifi-Sanjani M, Oyster N.M., et al. Cardiomyocyte-Specific Telomere Shortening is a Distinct Signature of Heart Failure in Humans. Journal of the American Heart Association. 2017;6:e005086
78. von Zglinicki T. Oxidative stress shortens telomeres. Trends Biochem Sci. 2002;27:339–344.

oxidative stress using antioxidants should be able to lengthen the telomeres. Experimental evidence shows this to be true. For example, lifestyle changes increased telomerase activity and reduced telomere length in a major study by the famed Dr. Dean Ornish in patients with prostate cancer.[79] I see no reason why heart disease patients would be any different. These are exciting times, and the future is in our hands.

---

79. Ornish, D., et al. Effect of comprehensive lifestyle changes on telomerase activity and telomere length in men with biopsy-proven low-risk prostate cancer: 5-year follow-up of a descriptive pilot study. The Lancet Oncology. Volume 14, No. 11, p1112–1120, October 2013.

SECTION 2

PREVENT

CHAPTER 12

PREVENT

Don't hate the players, hate the game.

Now that you understand (or hopefully should understand, after reading the previous 11 chapters), what some of the major *"players"* are—namely, your inherent *genetic risks*, as well as a whole host of *environmental factors*, including smoking, drinking, and diet—that may, but are not guaranteed to, contribute to serious cardiovascular disease, such as a heart attack.

This is why I think the saying, "Don't hate the player(s), hate the game." makes a lot of sense. In other words, the point is not to just focus solely on hating your lot in life if you were "dealt a bad hand," e.g., if you have a few genetic risk factors, and you work at a high-stress job. That is *hating the players*, and really will not get you too far, because the *game* is really the *Game of Life* and requires you to have an understanding and be flexible. The *Game* is whether you will have that heart attack or not.

- That said, we now have come to the point in our book where we have completed our overview of a good, representative variety of some of the important players in a heart attack.
- Now, we will use those assumptions, and others, and then take the next step: integrating the PREDICTIONS, assumptions, and clinical data to create customized recommendations so we can help you (and other similarly situated patients) to **PREVENT a heart attack**.

LIFESTYLE

The Cardiology culture is still a Fix-It culture.[80] This will need to change. Instead of fixing the damage, we need to use PREDICTIVE, PREVENTING and PIONEERING tools to prevent the damage.

"Minimally invasive" is still major surgery—and the cardiology community is still geared toward fixing the problem after the fact, not before the damage is done! With the method I have developed in my own practice, I am giving my patients the tools to PREDICT their chances of a heart attack within the next few years. Some of you might say, "I'm scared! I don't want to know." Well, that's a bunch of baloney! I am betting my entire company and my professional reputation on the simple proposition that you absolutely *would* want to know what your risk of suffering a heart attack was, **if** you knew you could meaningfully mitigate that risk by taking some simple supplements, medications, or even changing your **lifestyle factors**, and by "meaningfully mitigate that risk," I mean actually **change the odds so they were in** *your favor.* And that's the whole reason I'm writing, and you're reading, this book.

Lifestyle Factors **can make huge differences in preventing overall progression of heart disease and diabetes, meaning lower all-cause mortality and fewer heart attacks.**

---

80. By that, I mean, most of the profession is geared toward treatment, and mainly surgical treatment: Even medical treatment (pills) takes a back seat to cutting and "Roto-Rootering" out the visible and obvious problem, which feels more practical and final. Prevention just is not as "exciting" to most cardiology practitioners, and certainly not those who are cardiac surgeons.

The truth is that people from our *grandparents' generation* seemed to know a lot more about this than we give them credit for. As proof, I offer the following huge hit from 1929:

1. *Button up your overcoat,*
   When the wind is free,
   Take good care of yourself,
   You belong to me!
2. *Oh, eat an apple every day,*
   Get to bed by three,
   Oh, take good care of yourself,
   You belong to me!
3. *Be careful crossing streets, ooh-ooh,*
   Cut out sweets, ooh-ooh,
   Lay off meats, ooh-ooh,
   You'll get a pain and ruin your tum-tum!
4. *Beware of frozen ponds, ooh-ooh,*
   Stocks and bonds, ooh-ooh,
   Peroxide blondes, ooh-ooh,
   You'll get a pain and ruin your bankroll!
5. *Keep the spoon out of your cup,*
   When you're drinking tea,
   Oh, take good care of yourself,
   You belong to me!

Songwriters: B.G. DESYLVA, LEW BROWN, RAY HENDERSON
Button Up Your Overcoat lyrics © 1928 Warner/Chappell Music, Inc.,
RAY HENDERSON MUSIC CO., INC.

THE BIG 3 LIFESTYLE FACTORS

1. Diet
2. Exercise
3. Stress Reduction

1.   DIET

As any cardiologist worth his salt will tell you, diet is perhaps the *definitive* lifestyle solution—but only if you stick to it, which, of course, few patients do.

The Entrenched Problem

Diets based only on Counting Calories, Drinking Diet Sodas, and Low Fat/Low-Cholesterol Diets are the Wrong Way to Go for Better Heart Health! Please STOP!

It is my sincere hope that if you have gotten this far in reading this book, you will understand *why* all of those diets are not going to make you lose weight consistently, nor will they prevent you from getting a heart attack or other cardiovascular disease; in fact, they are harmful.

The conclusion is inescapable: the only two diets that have consistently been shown to be successful in lowering rates of cardiovascular disease are the "Mediterranean diet." and "The plant-based diet."

WHAT IS THE MEDITERRANEAN DIET?

The term "Mediterranean Diet" has become subject to a wide variety of interpretations, some of them wildly incorrect. Usually, people like to say that the Mediterranean Diet has lots of olive oil from Italy and Greece, and also fresh fish, which also are plentiful from the Mediterranean Sea. While not a meatless diet, beef is de-emphasized, as the local cultures in those countries tended to eat predominantly lamb and poultry. Dairy products, when served, are always full-fat, never low-fat or skim. Fresh fruits and vegetables are always served liberally. Grains are always true whole grains, never refined. Sweets are kept to a minimum. Wine is an integral part of meals. Portions are moderate. However, that is still just vague.

There is one, single Mediterranean Diet. Different countries in the Mediterranean have different variations on the dietary theme. I, for example, don't encourage red meat. Even lamb is red meat. I explained why earlier: because red meat creates TMAO, which is an oxidant. Oxidants are not good for your blood vessels. As an example, I like to look to an actual study[81] that defined the term, and got results.

In the study, the Mediterranean Diet group received the following diet recommendations:

Mediterranean Diet

Food	Goal
Recommended	
Olive oil (extra-virgin, polyphenol-rich, (includes amounts used in cooking, salads.)	≥ 4 tbsp/day (Qty for MD+EVOO)
Tree nuts and peanuts	≥ 3 servings/wk (Qty for MD+ Nuts)
Fresh fruits	≥ 3 servings/day
Vegetables	≥ 2 servings/day
Sofrito*	≥ 2 servings/wk
Fish (esp. fatty fish), seafood	≥ 3 servings/wk
Legumes	≥ 3 servings/wk
White meat	Instead of red meat
Wine with meals (optional, only for habitual drinkers)	≥ 7 glasses/wk
Discouraged	
Soda drinks	< 1 drink/day
Commercial** bakery goods, sweets, pastries	< 3 servings/wk
"Spread fats" i.e., butter or margarine	< 1 serving/day
Red and processed meats	< 1 serving/day

* Sofrito is a sauce made with tomato, onion, garlic and herbs, simmered with olive oil, popular in Spanish cookery.

** "Commercial bakery goods, sweets, pastries" (not homemade) including cakes, cookies, biscuits, and custard.

Now, for those of you who haven't recognized this by now, you should immediately be saying, "But Dr. B.,what about the *control group*, what diet did they get?" Well, I'm glad you asked, because, for every study group, there is obviously a control group

81. Estruch R, Ros E, Salas-Salvado, J, et al. Primary Prevention of Cardiovascular Disease with a Mediterranean Diet Supplemented with Extra-Virgin Olive Oil or Nuts. (June 21, 2018) N Engl J Med 2018; 378:e34

against which the study group must be measured, and for these investigators, it was the standard "low-fat" diet that mainstream cardiologists have been recommending for years. Nice target, guys.

And here's what that control group's dietary recommendations were:

Low-Fat Diet Control Group

Food	Goal
Recommended	
Low-fat dairy products	≥ 3 servings/day
Bread, potatoes, pasta, rice	≥ 3 servings/day
Fresh fruits	≥ 3 servings/day
Vegetables	≥ 2 servings/day
Lean fish and seafood	≥ 3 servings/wk
Discouraged	
Vegetable oils (including olive oil)	≤ 2 tbsp/day
Commercial bakery goods, sweets, pastries	≤ 1 serving/wk
"Nuts and fried snacks"	≤ 1 serving/wk
Red and processed fatty meats	≤ 1 serving/wk
Visible fat in meats and soups	Always remove
Fatty fish, seafood, canned in oil	≤ 1 serving/wk
Spread fats	≤ 1 serving/wk
Sofrito	≤ 2 servings/wk

I should clarify that this *particular study* actually broke participants into *three* groups: the Mediterranean Diet *with extra olive oil* group, the Mediterranean Diet *with nuts* group, and the control group *(the low-fat diet group)*. That didn't mean that people who regularly ate a Mediterranean Diet in other ways were not eating any olive oil, of course. They almost certainly were. They just weren't typically eating a minimum of 4 tablespoons a day, as the "MD + EVOO" group were advised to do. Similarly, with the "MD+Nuts" group: they were told to eat at least three servings per week of at least 30 grams per serving. My reason for including these tables is that it gives you a very good definition of a plan that you could reasonably follow.

I was already going to call this kind of diet the "Modified Mediterranean" because it omitted red meat. This study already did that. And the investigators and I did not even talk, I swear! But I like the way they did these tables, because they allow for the possibility that the study participants *might* eat as much as one serving of red meat per day, or three commercial bakery sweets per week, even a glass of soda a day.

Does the [Modified] Mediterranean Diet Really Work?

As they might say in Fargo, North Dakota, "Oh, you betcha!" A direct quote from the "Conclusions" section of the study I cited earlier states:

"In this study involving persons at high cardiovascular risk, the incidence of major cardiovascular events was lower among those assigned to a Mediterranean diet supplemented with extra-virgin olive oil or nuts than among those assigned to a reduced-fat diet." How much lower? For the "MD + EVOO" group, the hazard ratio (HR) was only 0.69, and for the "MD + nuts" group, the HR was 0.72 compared to the control group (HR=1.00). This means that those groups were only 69% and 72%, respectively, as likely to have a cardiovascular event as the low-fat control group.

Another thing that the data in both the Mediterranean groups and the low-fat control groups reveals is that, while the low-fat group's "recommended" list included *low-fat* dairy products, its "discouraged" list did not include *full-fat* dairy products. And, they are absent completely on the Mediterranean diet list, even though it is well known that inhabitants of Mediterranean countries ate dairy products: milk, cheese, yogurt, etc. However, they were all full-fat. My theory is that full-fat dairy products are either healthy, or are at least, not harmful. However, low-fat dairy products are harmful. This has been borne out by a number of studies: this is only the latest. However, as you can see, because there was no stated dietary proscription against it, the Mediterranean Diet groups may very well have been having full-fat dairy products yet been complying with the rest of the diet. After all, what is much of Mediterranean cuisine without cheese and yogurt?

WHAT IS A PLANT-BASED DIET?

Well simply put, a plant-based diet means consuming foods that are primarily from plants. Of course, this includes whole-grains, fruits and vegetables, but also beans, legumes, nuts, seeds, oils, spices, herbs and seasonings. Now, eating a plant-based diet doesn't mean that you only consume non-animal products, such as a strict vegan would. Nor does it mean that you never indulge in meat or dairy products. Instead, it just means the vast majority of the food you choose to consume on a daily basis should come from a plant source and not an animal source. But, vegetarian and vegan diets are still considered plant-based, they are just more strictly plant based. Vegetarian diets have been shown to support one's health by lowering their risk of developing CAD, high blood pressure and diabetes, as well as increasing longevity.[82]

The different types of Vegetarian diets:

1) Semi-vegetarian or flexitarian: consume eggs and dairy, but only on very few occasions do they consume meat, poultry, fish, and seafood.
2) Pescatarian: consume eggs, dairy, fish, and seafood, but do not consume any meat or poultry.
3) Vegetarian: consume eggs and dairy foods, but do not consume any meat, poultry, fish, or seafood.
4) Vegan: do not consume any animal foods whatsoever, including no eggs and no dairy.

People who eat plant-based diets, including vegetarian diets, can successfully consume all of the necessary protein, fats,

---

82. Kahleova, Hana, Levin, Susan, and Barnard, Neal (2017). Cardio-Metabolic Benefits of Plant-Based Diets, Nutrients, 9(8)848; doi:10.3390/nu9080848. http://www.mdpi.com/2072-6643/9/8/848

carbohydrates, vitamins, and minerals of a balanced diet needed for optimal health, and are often higher in fiber and phytonutrients. However, some vegans may need to take extra supplements to meet all of their nutritional needs, specifically vitamin B12, which is essential to health and can only be obtained through the consumption of animal products.

If you are limiting or cutting out animal products from your diet, well then technically, your diet will naturally also be lower in fat, cholesterol, and salt. We all know that diets high in salt, cholesterol and fat are associated with a higher risk of heart disease. So if you are cutting out most of these food sources from your diet, then does it also lower your chances of developing heart disease and/or a heart attack?

Well, for one, vegetarian diets have already been associated with a lowered risk for developing CVD in general, including coronary artery disease and cerebrovascular disease (ex. stroke). Other common heart disease risk factors are also seen less frequently in vegetarians. In the European Prospective Investigation into Cancer and Nutrition study, vegetarians had a 32% lower risk of developing coronary heart disease, compared with non-vegetarians. The Lifestyle Heart Trial found that 82% of patients diagnosed with heart disease who followed this plant-based diet program had some level of regression of atherosclerosis and 91% had a reduction in the frequency of angina episodes. In addition, the study showed a 37.2% reduction in LDL that is similar to results achieved with lipid-lowering medications.[83] The more recent literature is now suggesting that changing your diet to a mostly plant-based diet may not only help prevent CAD, but also reverse it.

It's well established that atherosclerosis (plaque build up) is

---

83. Dean Ornish, Larry W. Scherwitz, James H. Billings, K. Lance Gould, Terri A. Merritt, Stephen Sparler, William T. Armstrong, Thomas A. Ports, Richard L. Kirkeeide, Charissa Hogeboom, Richard J. Brand, (1998). Intensive Lifestyle Changes for Reversal of Coronary Heart Disease, JAMA, 280(23), 2001-2007. doi: http://dx.doi.org/10.1001/jama.280.23.2001.

associated with diets high in meat, fat, and carbohydrates. As I discussed in the previous chapters, atherosclerosis results from slow, progressive damage to the endothelial cells that line the inner walls of blood vessels that eventually results in an increase in endothelial dysfunction. Furthermore, certain metabolites of L-carnitine, for example trimethylamine-N-oxide (TMAO), are produced as a result of consuming red meat and have been recently identified as a novel predictive biomarker of coronary artery disease (CAD). And that's because researchers discovered that the metabolism of L-carnitine by the intestinal microbiome is only associated with higher amounts of atherosclerosis in omnivores. Whereas vegetarians do not have this same negative metabolic effect, which is one of the reasons why a plant-based diet is now associated with a lower risk of CAD. By replacing some of your red meat consumption with more plant foods, you are reducing the ability of TMAO to cause injury and damage to your endothelial cells. Therefore, reducing the amount of damage that can cause endothelial dysfunction and increase the formation of plaque build up.[84]

On top of reducing the circulation of factors that are known to be injurious to endothelial cells, plant-based foods also provide a protective effect against atherosclerosis by increasing the circulation of certain endothelial protective factors. Polyphenols are a type of chemical compound that make up a group of over 500 different phytochemicals, which are a type of micronutrients that occur naturally in plants. These are what give plants their beautiful color, but they also help plants protect themselves from various environmental dangers. When consuming plant products, you are also absorbing different types of polyphenols depending on the plant source and they can act as powerful antioxidants. Experts believe that when we consume these plant-derived compounds, we also get some of the protective effects. In particular, they help prevent our vascular endothelial cells from

---

84. Tuso, P., Stoll, S. R., & Li, W. W. (2015). A plant-based diet, atherogenesis, and coronary artery disease prevention. The Permanente journal, 19(1), 62-7; doi: 10.7812/TPP/14-036. https://www.ncbi.nlm.nih.gov/pmc/articles/PMC4315380/

damage due to oxidative stress by preventing the oxidation of LDL-C (the "bad" cholesterol).[85]

In general, compared to the individuals who frequently consume red meat, people who tend to consume less red meat and eat more vegetables have a lower body mass index (a weight-to-height ratio that is used to classify individuals as underweight, normal weight, or overweight), lower systolic blood pressure, lower serum levels of LDL-C, and thinner blood vessel intimal medial wall thickness. And compared to an omnivore diet, a heavily plant-based diet is shown to result in less oxidative stress and less inflammation. The three main proposed mechanisms for how a plant-based diet may prevent atherosclerosis and CAD events are:

1) Prevention of VEC injury by eating foods low in sugar, salt, and fat.
2) Prevention of LDL oxidation by increased intake of fresh fruits and vegetables containing polyphenols.
3) Prevention of macrophage activation by decreasing intake of red meat, by exercise, and by stress reduction.[86]

A plant-based diet has been shown to help prevent and even treat Type 2 diabetes by significantly reducing HbA1c levels and improving blood sugar control. Compared to conventional diets used to treat Type 2 diabetes, a vegetarian diet can be almost twice as effective. Completely eliminating meat, cheese, and eggs is likely to lead to further improvements in body weight, glycemic

---

85. Wenlong Jianga, Huabing Weib, and Ben Hea (2015). Dietary flavonoids intake and the risk of coronary heart disease: A dose-response meta-analysis of 15 prospective studies, Thrombosis Research, 135(3):459-463. doi:10.1016/j.thromres.2014.12.016. https://www.sciencedirect.com/science/article/pii/S0049384814006859

86. Tuso, P., Stoll, S. R., & Li, W. W. (2015). A plant-based diet, atherogenesis, and coronary artery disease prevention. The Permanente journal, 19(1), 62-7; doi: 10.7812/TPP/14-036. https://www.ncbi.nlm.nih.gov/pmc/articles/PMC4315380/

control, and blood lipid levels.[87] Plant-based diets have also been shown to reduce insulin resistance and platelet aggregation.

Since dietary cholesterol is only found in animal products, it makes sense that omitting these from your diet will result in significant reductions in total and LDL cholesterol, which in turn also reduces your risk of heart disease. Switching to vegetarian diet has been shown to have a similar effect to that of statin therapy on improvement fasting and postprandial blood lipids.[88]

Not all Plant-Based Diets are Equal

The research is clear when it comes to associating a plant-based diet with a lower risk of heart disease. But do all of the different types of plant-based diets have the same positive effect? And do you really have to take drastic measures and cut out all sources of meat from your diet? Well, it's not that I don't agree with the benefits of a vegetarian diet, but rather I don't expect my patients to just quit meat cold turkey. What I do tell them is that moderation is key. And for your heart's sake, it's important to focus on the quantity of animal foods and the quality of plant foods. Let me explain what I mean. By just reducing your consumption of animal foods, it's still possible to reap the health benefits without completely eliminating them from your diet.

By limiting the quantity of animal products, it's thought to down-regulate the atherogenesis inflammatory initiation process by

---

87. Mishra, S., Xu, J., Agarwal, U., Gonzales, J., Levin, S., & Barnard, N. D. (2013). A multicenter randomized controlled trial of a plant-based nutrition program to reduce body weight and cardiovascular risk in the corporate setting: the GEICO study. European journal of clinical nutrition, 67(7), 718-24; doi: 10.1038/ejcn.2013.92. https://www.ncbi.nlm.nih.gov/pmc/articles/pmid/23695207/

88. Agnieszka Kuchta, Anna Lebiedzińska, Marcin Fijałkowski, Rafał Gałąska, Ewelina Kreft, Magdalena Totoń, Kuba Czaja, Anna Kozłowska, Agnieszka Ćwiklińska, Barbara Kortas-Stempak, Adrian Strzelecki, Anna Gliwińska, Kamil Dąbkowski, Maciej Jankowski, (2016). Impact of plant-based diet on lipid risk factors for atherosclerosis, Cardiology Journal, 23(2):141-148; doi: 10.5603/CJ.a2016.0002. https://journals.viamedica.pl/cardiology_journal/article/view/43847

decreasing the intake of substances found in processed foods, added sugars, oils, and meats that promote atherogenesis. And increasing the quantity of quality plant based products, is more likely to initiate the reciprocal increased intake of bioactive substances found in plants that protect the endothelium and inhibit atherogenesis. If I choose to limit my animal food consumption and replace it with a diet that mainly consists of processed and sugary foods, it would still be considered plant-based. However, this is not going to give you the same benefits that I described above and might even be worse for your health. If someone just eats junk food (chips, donuts, etc.) all day, they are not consuming the "more healthy" plant foods compared to "less-healthy" plant foods (juices/sweetened beverages, refined grains, potatoes/fries, sweets) and animal foods.

A diet mainly consisting of "healthy" plant foods (whole grains, fruits/vegetables, nuts/legumes, oils, tea/coffee) means a diet higher in dietary fiber, antioxidants, unsaturated fat and micronutrient content, and low in saturated fat and heme iron content, all of which could aid in weight loss/maintenance, enhance glycemic control and insulin regulation, improve lipid profile, reduce blood pressure, improve vascular health, decrease inflammation, and foster more favorable diet-gut microbiome interactions (through lowered levels of TMAO), thereby lowering CHD risk.

Dr. Satija headed a very insightful study that was published in the Journal of the American College of Cardiology in July 25, 2017. It tracked the diets of 209,000 adults for over two decades in order to compare three different types of plant-based diets with heart disease risk.
- Group 1 was an overall plant-based diet that emphasized consumption of all healthy plant foods while reducing intake of all animal foods, like dairy (skim, low-fat, and whole milk; cream, ice cream, yogurt, and cheese), eggs, fish, meat (chicken, turkey, beef, and pork), and foods that contain animal products like pizza, soups, and mayonnaise.

- Group 2 was a healthful plant-based diet that emphasized consumption of only healthy plant foods, such as whole grains, fruits, vegetables, nuts, legumes, and healthy oils, while reducing intake of less healthy plant foods as well as animal foods.
- Group 3 was an unhealthful plant-based diet that emphasized consumption of less healthy plant foods, such as fruit juices, refined grains (pasta, white rice, and processed breads and cereals), potatoes (French fries and potato chips), and sugar-sweetened beverages, while reducing the intake of healthy plant foods as well as animal foods. No surprise, they found that the people who followed the healthy plant-based diet (the second group) had the lowest risk for heart disease. They were also more active and leaner. On the other hand, those who followed the unhealthful plant-based diet (the third group) had a substantially higher risk for heart disease.

Thus, the study found that reducing animal foods doesn't necessarily lead to a healthier diet and greater heart protection if the resulting diet is based on less healthy plant foods. While this study didn't look at which animal foods, especially meat, could have an impact on heart health, other research has shown that, as with plant foods, the type and amount matter most.

Just four weeks of eating a "healthy" plant-based diet can result in significant clinical reductions in lipids and both systolic and diastolic blood pressure, as well as blood pressure medication usage. Statistically significant reductions were also observed for other CVD risk factors, including body weight, heart rate, waist circumference, insulin, HbA1c, and hs-CRP. This intervention demonstrated that a plant-based diet can be used effectively in the clinical setting with profound results.[89]

---

89. Richter, C. K., Skulas-Ray, A. C., Champagne, C. M., & Kris-Etherton, P. M. (2015). Plant protein and animal proteins: do they differentially affect cardiovascular disease risk?. Advances in nutrition (Bethesda, Md.), 6(6), 712-28. doi:10.3945/an.115.009654

However, not all plant-based diets are equal. White rice and white bread are plant-based foods, but you have read the previous chapters and you know they are not good for you. To keep your energy levels up and help you feel healthy in the long term, your diet needs to feed more than your stomach. It has to satiate your muscles, which crave protein; your digestive system, which runs best with fiber; and your tissues and bones, which work optimally when they're getting vitamins from food. A combination of whole grains, fruits, vegetables, proteins, and fats accomplishes that goal. This balance is also key to keeping you full after a meal and energized throughout the day so you don't feel the need to overeat.

Back to the Harvard Study: The Plant-Based Mediterranean Diet

The key to health and longevity is a diet rich in vegetables, proteins (this is where the debate of plant-based proteins vs. animal-based proteins comes in), and healthy fats, while also low in trans fat, heavily processed foods, refined carbohydrates like white bread, and sugary sweets and desserts. Don't worry meat lovers. You don't have to completely cut out animal products from your diet. It's not realistic for most and it's not completely necessary. But, you do need to try to limit your consumption, especially when it comes to red meat. Focus on lean meat and poultry when you can. And try to save that delicious steak for special occasions. Now the main reason I recommend a Mediterranean diet that's more plant-based than animal-based is because the Mediterranean diet focuses on good, healthy fats, which are essential. What's interesting about this study is that participants didn't always eat healthy; in fact, they started increasing their intake of plant-based foods in middle age. And the healthy plant foods still increased their longevity, while processed foods and sugary drinks lowered it.

The focus should be on eating more of the right plants, avoiding the wrong kind, eliminating unhealthy foods, and moderating your intake of healthier animal products. A heart-healthy diet doesn't need to be daunting either.For instance, replace white rice with brown rice or other whole grains, and white bread with whole-grain bread. Choose oatmeal instead of processed cereal, and water instead of juice drinks. If embracing a full plant-based diet feels intimidating, then begin small. "A moderate change in your diet, such as lowering your animal food intake by one to two servings per day and replacing it with legumes or nuts as your protein source, can have a lasting positive impact on your health,"

A Modified Mediterranean Diet, and what the above study is calling the Mediterranean Diet, supplemented with extra virgin olive oil and nuts, is the only proven and the most effective diet to prevent and reduce cardiovascular disease and heart attack. It is even more effective if it can be tailor-made to each individual patient based on his/her individual genetics and makeup.

2. EXERCISE

You probably have heard the statistic that well over a third of Americans are overweight or obese. It's sad but true. Part of the reason, no doubt, is that we overeat, and we are eating the wrong kinds of food. Another part of the reason is that we don't exercise enough. But, apart from the fact that exercise helps us to lose weight, exercise is important because it keeps us from being sedentary. Yes, that was meant to be obvious. But sitting still was not meant to be our ordinary state of affairs. We were meant to be active creatures, and the more we don't move, the less healthy we are. Many studies have linked a sedentary lifestyle to a shortened lifespan. The American College of Cardiology currently recommends we do 45 minutes to an hour of some sort of exercise per day. However, this feels unrealistic for most people, many of my patients included: there just doesn't seem to be enough time in the day to devote to that amount of exercise. So, discouraged, they end up giving up, and not doing it at all. I also have a number of patients who actually have the exercise equipment in their homes, but don't seem to know how to use it, so they don't use it at all.

Getting Started

I understand that the recommendations of one hour a day seem daunting. Especially if you are deconditioned. Start with a short walk. If you have a dog, maybe that part has already been handled for you. The dog makes you take a walk (or two) for at least a short portion of the day. Let him or her be your walking buddy and go for five minutes more the next day. When your dog comes in, he/she may want a drink of water. You probably will too, but even if you don't want one, drink a glass of water anyway; now you'll both be hydrated. You'll feel exhausted at first, but it *will* get easier. If you don't have a dog, you *could* try it with your cat, but make sure you have a good harness on her, and I make no guarantees. Some cats like to walk on a leash. If you have no pets, your wife/husband/girlfriend/boyfriend/friend/neighbor is an excellent choice to accompany you. Especially if they have health concerns too. You will motivate each other.

All Cardio Is Not the Answer

When you do get on an exercise program—and you must—you should not do cardio exclusively. You should do cardio, of course, but you should also do a little bit of strength training. (Now, when I say "strength training," I don't mean bodybuilding like competitive weightlifters—I simply mean building muscle.) And I'm telling you this as a *cardiologist!* The term "skinny fat" is referred to people who lose significant weight doing only cardio without strength training as even though they look skinny, their body's fat to muscle ratio is high. Why is this important? Well, first of all, as you get older, you will lose muscle. Many studies have correlated muscle loss with decreased longevity. Low muscle mass makes you susceptible to infection, cancer and heart disease. It also reduces your metabolism and can predispose you to diabetes. People who have less muscle reserve are less likely to have the overall strength to survive a hospital admission. That's just a fact. So, weight training, done slowly and moderately, allows you to gain muscle. Then, as you adapt to it, you can make it a part of an **interval training** regimen, wherein you alternate back and forth between cardio (high-intensity) and weight training (low-intensity) activities. This allows you to get a more effective workout, and, according to one study, it has specific utility with patients who have coronary artery disease.[90] I have seen patients who have treadmills just gathering dust, not sure how to use them, especially if they have been out of shape for a long time. I tell them a very simple rule to remember: Keep it moderate, you're not running a marathon. Try to do the treadmill with someone nearby and sing or talk to them. They should be able to hear and understand you. If they don't, you're doing too much! Turn the speed down.

We used to think the more strenuous the exercise, the better for our health. That's why boot camps were created. Recent studies, however, have shown that strenuous exercise or any prolonged and constant stress on your body, be it in the form of a boot camp or running a marathon not only is not beneficial, but negatively affects your health and longevity. Even though these studies came as a surprise, it does make sense. Extreme stress causes the release of stress hormones and increases your sympathetic nervous system activity on a chronic basis, both of which, as you learned in the previous chapters, can be detrimental to your health. So next time, you decided to sign up for the boot camp at your gym I suggest you look for other alternatives.

3. STRESS REDUCTION

I have talked to you extensively in Chapter 9 about how mental/emotional stress directly causes cardiovascular disease, such as heart attack and stroke. This means it is

---

90. Cornish, Aimee K.; Broadbent, Suzanne; Cheema, Birinder S. (23 October 2010). "Interval training for patients with coronary artery disease: a systematic review." European Journal of Applied Physiology. 111 (4): 579–589.

crucial that you take whatever steps are necessary to reduce that stress. Some of the stressors, for example, life events that are unexpected, such as loved ones passing away, may not be stressors you can reduce. However, you can try to reduce stress related to your personal and family relationships, your work life, and other things which are somewhat in your control. Sometimes, simply talking things out helps, even to a therapist, because when you feel that you can't talk about your problems to anyone, those feelings become more and more upsetting if the underlying situation continues unchanged, leading to greater stress.

Some people find that yoga, t'ai chi, or meditation are practices that reduce overall stress by refocusing people on other things than the stressors, as well as diminishing the physical manifestation of stress. Sometimes, certain medications, such as alpha blockers, may help reduce these physical manifestations of stress as well, making patients more able to deal with everyday life. These medications may also be beneficial to certain cardiac patients as well.

However you do it, reducing stress is a must in order to enjoy life on the path to live to be a 100.

CHAPTER 13

MEDICATION VS. SUPPLEMENTS, NUTRACEUTICALS AND MEDICAL FOODS

In my nearly twenty years of medical practice, I find that there has been a constant source of confusion about the role of medications and supplements among my patients: Where do I stand? Where should I stand? As an integrative medicine practitioner, should I not automatically decry the evils of Big Pharma and shout them from the highest mountaintops? I will try to explain what my positions are, and why.

I. "Do I Really Need to Take Medications, Dr. B?"

This is, perhaps, one of the most common questions I get from new patients, who often come to me knowing that I am an integrative cardiologist, i.e., a cardiologist who combines conventional as well as more natural approaches, including supplements, nutraceuticals and medical foods, to treat cardiac disease. So, they often come to me, [multiple] medication bottles in hand, expecting me to tell them just to throw them out the window because I have a magic elixir of herbs, or a combination of supplements, that can fully replace them. The most common medication most people who see me want to stop is the statin family of medications.

There is not a day that I don't get at least two patients who either see me wanting me to replace their Lipitor or Crestor for something more natural, or they just refuse to take this medication. Even though some of these requests can be safely and reliably granted, the benefit of taking these medications far outweighs the risks.

The advent of HMG Co-A reductase inhibitors (what we call statins) in the 1980s significantly reduced the incidence of heart attacks, the morbidity associated with heart attacks, and effectively reduced the chances of a second heart attack. Over the past three decades, numerous large randomized double-blinded studies involving hundreds of thousands of patients have confirmed these findings. There is absolutely no doubt the statins, if used in the RIGHT GROUP OF PATIENTS, can be extremely effective in preventing heart attacks. However, the key here is the "RIGHT GROUP OF PATIENTS." Let me explain further. Physicians in the 1980s and 1990s, seeing these impressive results, started putting almost every patient with even the slightest elevation in cholesterol on these medications. Physicians themselves, without any risk factors for heart disease, started taking these medications preemptively to PREVENT heart attacks. As one of my colleagues put it nicely: "doctors put these medications in water supplies."

It became common after the 1990s to see healthy individuals (with no risk factors for heart disease) in their early thirties taking statins as prescribed by their primary physicians, just because their cholesterol was slightly elevated.

Statins, however, as everyone knows these days, come with some unpleasant side effects (just like any medication). Even though the side effects are not life-threatening in most cases (unless you don't check your liver function regularly, have pre-existing liver or muscle disease and /or overdose on it), the non-life threatening side effects could be severe in some patients. The most common side effect is muscle ache, muscle tenderness, or in some cases muscle weakness. They frequently cause fatigue. They block the production of stress hormones, sex hormones, and Vitamin D, as well as Coenzyme Q which is important for efficient functioning of our cells, especially in our muscle, brain, heart, liver and skin tissues. More importantly, recent research has indicated that chronic use of statins can increase the development of diabetes in susceptible patients. [N.B. The concern for development of dementia and cancer was put to rest after multiple studies failed to show any relationship].

Given the common and bothersome risk factors of this group of medications, coupled with overuse/ misuse in groups of patients who would not benefit from it, more and more practitioners (mostly naturopathic and holistic practitioners) started to create a negative campaign against these medications. Soon the "horrible, dangerous" side effects filled the media and different websites and blogs.

So at the present moment, a war is raging between the conventional medical community and the naturopathic/ holistic community in regards to the use of statins. The naturopathic community views stains as priests view evil and hold a cross to ward off the evil. The word statin is prohibited in many "alternative and holistic" clinics and all the world problems and disasters are attributed to these medications, whereas in conventional medical and cardiology clinics, statins are the holy grail for prevention and treatment of most heart diseases (coronary heart disease). The solution here again lies in the adoption of an integrative approach (what we call the B-100 method in our clinic). Let me explain.

In understanding the solution, first you have to understand that the practice of Medicine involves balancing the risks vs. the benefits. I have to balance the risk vs. the benefit of each and every treatment for every single patient of mine on a daily basis, and make sure that:

1) this is the best treatment possible
2) that the benefit outweighs the risk and
3) that the risk is not substantial

So when it comes to deciding if a patient really needs to be on a statin, the same decision-making algorithm applies: Statins have only shown to provide benefit in the following group of patients:

1. Patients with a prior history of a heart attack, or a history of coronary angioplasty/stent or a history of CABG surgery.
2. A very strong family (first-degree family) history of premature coronary artery disease (younger than 55 in men and 65 in women).
3. History of stroke.
4. A history of long-established diabetes.
5. Very high levels of bad cholesterol (LDL > 190) which is deemed to be familial (Familial hypercholesterolemia).
6. Elevated calcium score on CT coronary calcium scan.

Therefore, if you don't fit into any of the above categories, you do not need and should not be on statins. So then, does it mean if you don't have any of the above conditions you don't have to worry about your cholesterol levels? Well, you still do. The problem is that most practitioners are not educated or knowledgable on how to reduce cholesterol levels naturally. Medical schools don't teach you natural remedies and don't talk much about supplements. I remember in my entire medical school training, only one very small chapter (a few pages) was dedicated to natural supplements or vitamins! So faced with the challenge of lowering their patient's cholesterol levels (after the patient fails diet and exercise and weight loss, these doctors either prescribe the only thing they know, or just choose to ignore the high cholesterol levels. There are, however, many natural and effective remedies to lower the cholesterol, many of which I utilize in my program.

Patient Case:

A.H. was a 38-year-old male executive who came to see me for a second opinion in regards to his medications. He had been noted to have "high cholesterol" by his primary physician who started him on Lipitor (Atorvastatin) about six months prior. The patient noted severe leg cramps many nights, waking him up from sleep. He decided to see a cardiologist as a second opinion who switched him to Crestor (Rosuvastatin). Even though his leg cramps were resolved, he noted severe fatigue which was interfering with his daily activities. The cardiologist then reduced the dose of the medication which didn't help. The primary doctor then switched him to Zocor (simvastatin) which caused muscle aches and liver enzyme abnormalities.

Frustrated, he came to see me. I determined that he had no risk factors for coronary heart disease. I then referred him for a CT calcium scan which showed no calcification in his coronary arteries. Therefore, it was obvious to me that he should not have ever been placed on statin therapy to begin with. He was very relieved and happy to know he didn't need to be on statins. I then started him on a combination of Bergamot, Berberine and plant sterols. His blood test three months after using these supplements had reached the desirable levels without any side effects. At his last office visit, he was feeling great and thankful.

(1) When is it not wishful thinking?

If you are among the few patients whose conditions, such as diabetes, or high blood pressure, are mild enough that they can truly be controlled by lifestyle factors alone (diet, exercise, and stress reduction), you may actually be able to ditch the medications you have been using to control those conditions. But everybody thinks they could be among that group, so I would really have to examine your individual case closely and carefully before making that determination. If your condition is mild, you might be able to control those conditions using carefully selected vitamins and supplements along with a healthy diet, exercise and perhaps weight loss. Otherwise, can some of these patients **reduce the dosage** of their existing medications, or **cut out** some of their existing medications?

(2) **The answer is dependent on the individual patient's condition, but often, the answer is YES.**
First of all, I need to disabuse you of a lot of myths about so-called "holistic practitioners" and how they view conventional medications. Let me begin by saying that even the *word* "holistic" has been corrupted; it means "whole," i.e., encompassing everything, which is what I do as an *integrative* medicine practitioner. Here's a misconception among many patients. Even many self-described "holistic" practitioners will use conventional medications: for example, if they see a patient who is pre-diabetic, but dangerously close to diabetic, they may prescribe metformin to lower the patient's A1C levels, even though the official guidelines don't yet call for it. However, they may also add natural remedies, such as cinnamon, berberine, and turmeric, to the mix, which also have been proven to be potent at lowering blood glucose. If their patient has borderline kidney disease, or their heart shows signs of working too hard, they may prescribe an ACE inhibitor. Even though the medications are "conventional," these practitioners are trying to head off further damage at the pass and realize that these medications have been proven safe and effective at preventing diabetes (in the first example) and kidney or heart disease (in the second example). I know as an integrative cardiologist, I do both of these things in my own practice.

So, what do I tell the patient whose conditions are not mild enough to be able to go completely off of their medications but still want me to replace their prescriptions with holistic alternatives, i.e., supplements? I tell them I can't usually do a complete replacement, but I can usually reduce the doses of the prescription medications they are taking. And how do I do this? I prescribe supplements in addition to their medications!

You see, I am typically against using high doses of many medications, especially the medications we have to use in the practice of cardiology, such as antihypertensives, a.k.a. blood-pressure medications, particularly diuretics, such as hydrochlorothiazide or furosemide (Lasix) and blood thinners, such as warfarin, which often have difficult to intolerable side effects, as well as narrow therapeutic indices. (What is a narrow therapeutic index? It means there is very little margin between the effective dose and a lethal dose, but some have expanded that term to include the margin between the effective dose and a dose that causes intolerable side effects.)

YOU'RE NOT JUST GETTING OLD: MEDICATION CONSIDERATIONS FOR SENIORS

Many patients complain of severe exhaustion, or depression, thinking that they must be just getting old. Well, it turns out, more than once, the problem is an overly high dose of a blood-pressure medication—which had fatigue as a major side effect, and which elderly patients may be more sensitive to—because their kidneys are not as able to clear the metabolites of the drug as quickly out of their bodies as are younger patients. Add to this the pervasive issue of "polypharmacy," the typically large number of other medications that seniors are commonly prescribed, which have side effects of their own, which often compound the problem and may have drug interactions that went unidentified by other physicians or pharmacists, and it is no wonder that we have seen an increase in falls in elderly patients – they are often losing their balance because of medication side effects.

In many instances, it may be an issue of a medication whose dose may be standard for a 40-year-old, 200-pound man, but too high for an 80-year-old, 90-pound woman, whose kidneys cannot adequately clear the medication from her system, especially combined with other medications, which may potentiate (make stronger/increase) that medication's blood level. In cases like these, I am often able to reduce these patients' medication doses so that their medical problems are still treated effectively by adding supplements. You can get the maximum therapeutic effect out of the medication at a lower dose. This is a very significant issue in elderly patients.

Supplements can:

1) promote better absorption of the medication.
2) promote synergistic effects of the medication.
3) ameliorate side effects of medications.
4) possibly enable you to be treated with lower doses of the medication.
5) because of #1 to #4, possibly enable you to use less of the medication, generally speaking.

Because side effects are dose-dependent, you see fewer side effects by lowering the dose of the drug.

II. Are Supplements a Sham. A Flim-Flam? Or should they be Your Jam?

Generally, we have viewed vitamin and mineral supplements (beyond saying that patients should use them if they are *deficient* in vitamins and minerals), with skepticism, if not downright derision. Scurvy, rickets, and pellagra are diseases of the third world, not America, where we have "enriched flour," orange juice, and balanced diets, so we may believe there is no need for us to add Vitamin C or B vitamins to our daily intake. If you get enough sunlight, there's no need for anybody to take Vitamin D supplements, and the studies that attempted to link Vitamin D deficiency to a host of ills like cardiovascular disease and cancer supposedly proved nothing. Skeptics like to say that Vitamin E has no beneficial effect at all, and Vitamin A is toxic.

First of all, I should clarify that "supplements" are not just vitamins and minerals, although that is the most popular concept of them. Fish oil is a supplement; so are cinnamon and turmeric, which you normally find on your spice rack. But they also have medicinal properties. Although many medications are made in the lab, still many others are *natural products*, whether it was the needles of the Chinese yew tree, which gave us the chemotherapy drug taxol; the flowers of the foxglove plant, which gave us the heart drug, digitalis; the cinchona bark, which gave us quinine to quell malaria; or even the bark of the white willow tree, which gave us salicin, a precursor to salicylic acid and aspirin— all were indisputably natural products which led to the discovery of mainstream medications.

Thus, it should come as no surprise that berberine, which is a natural product of the alkaloid class, could be more than just a "supplement," but actually real medication, just like its other famous alkaloid cousins – such as the belladonna alkaloids (hyoscyamine and scopolamine), morphine, colchicine (for treating gout), and atropine (useful for treating bradycardia, a very slow heartbeat, as well as some types of second-degree heart block). If that doesn't convince you that "supplements," which can include flowers, herbs, barks, and fish oils, as well as the familiar vitamins and minerals, should deserve equal consideration along with conventional medication, I don't know what will.

NOT ALL SUPPLEMENTS ARE CREATED EQUAL!

Unfortunately, over the years, many poor-quality supplements have flooded the market. When consumers have chosen to buy the cheapest supplements, they, unfortunately, have often gotten what they've paid for – supplements that were not produced in facilities that were compliant with Good Manufacturing Practices (GMP). Because of that, these "cheapo" supplements also often had no standardization between batches, so you might not have any consistency between one bottle and another in terms of the dose you got. This lack of standardization is one reason that many in the medical community do not trust the supplement community. They felt they could not be guaranteed a consistent dose of active ingredient in every pill every time. I, too, was aware of that concern, and made sure to seek out only the best suppliers who custom-made my formulations of all the various supplements I provide for my patients to my exacting specifications, in a laboratory that is cGMP-compliant and ISO-9001-certified. These are the only supplements that I personally recommend to my patients, because they have met my rigorous approval.

Furthermore, let me address the often-held beliefs of mainstream medical professionals who purport that most of these supplements don't work.

Well, when I said that not all supplements are created equal, I acknowledge that there has been lingering confusion that has caused misinformation about the lack of effectiveness of various supplements. For example:

Vitamin E: A number of years ago, it was widely reported that that supplementation with Vitamin E was not only not *healthy*, but that it could actually kill you—that is, it appeared to increase all-cause mortality rates.[91] However, the study has been criticized for several reasons, such as not considering common factors such as, for example, smoking, and excluding the administration of other drugs. Do you think that might make a difference? But, beyond that is another factor: the study only considered "Vitamin E" to mean "alpha-tocopherol," because that was considered the most important, and, in supplements, was often the only tocopherol supplied. In the cheaper supplements, "Vitamin E" meant "dl-alpha-tocopherol," which is a synthetic form of alpha-tocopherol. But recent research shows that the other tocopherols,

---

91. Miller E.R., Pastor-Barriuso R., Dalal D., Riemersma R.A., Appel L.J., Guallar E. Meta-analysis: High-dosage vitamin E supplementation may increase all-cause mortality. Ann. Intern. Med. 2005;142:37–46.

such as γ-tocopherol (γT), δ-tocopherol, often listed on the bottle as "mixed tocopherols," as well as the tocotrienols, such as γ-tocotrienol, have unique antioxidant and anti-inflammatory properties that are *superior* to those of alpha-tocopherol.[92] So, by only restricting the analysis to "alpha-tocopherol," it is not the form of the supplement that I or other integrative medicine practitioners recommend, or would ever recommend, and the published result is thus misleading.

R-LIPOIC ACID/ALPHA-LIPOIC ACID

Here's where a *lot* of my patients and friends have become *very* confused. They think that R-Lipoic Acid and Alpha-Lipoic Acid are different products, but they're not. I wish that the manufacturers would call it R-Alpha-Lipoic Acid to differentiate it from the plain old Alpha-Lipoic Acid, which may, in truth, be (RS)-Lipoic Acid, which is known as racemic lipoic acid, or a 50/50 mixture of R- and S-Lipoic Acid. What do these R's and S's mean? Well, you have to believe me when I tell you that molecules, including lipoic acid molecules, can be right- or left-handed, and just suspend your disbelief. Just accept it.

These right or left-handed versions are called isomers. (See Fig.2, on following page.) This is important because R-Lipoic Acid has a much greater biological activity, and it is thought that the R-isomer is what exists in nature. So, if you buy "Alpha Lipoic Acid," you get a mixture of the R- and S-isomers, which may not get you the best result.

---

92. Jiang Q. Free Radic Biol Med. 2014 Jul;72:76-90. Natural forms of vitamin E: metabolism, antioxidant, and anti-inflammatory activities and their role in disease prevention and therapy.

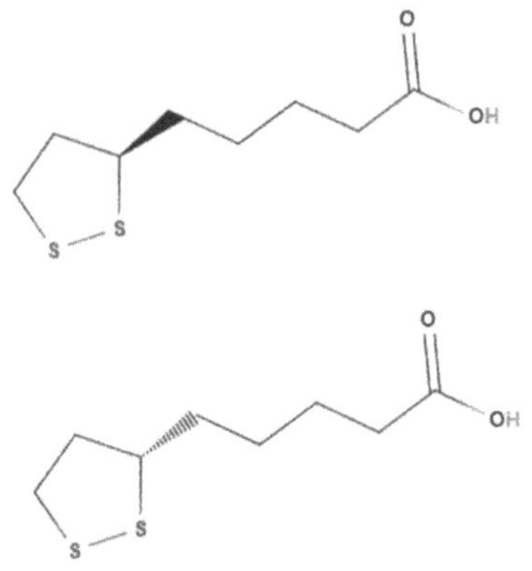

Fig. 2. At top, R-Lipoic Acid. Notice "wedge" coming out of pentagon, out of paper. At bottom, its stereochemical isomer, S-Lipoic Acid, whose wedge is going back into plane of paper. (Courtesy of NotoriousPyro, Licensed by Creative Commons.)

Reasons like this are why I do my part to educate my patients. Because I believe when you fully understand what there is to know about supplements, you will agree with me that they are a powerful adjunct to conventional medical treatment that can only strengthen the effectiveness of that treatment, while reducing any negatives associated with it.

CHAPTER 14

NUTRACEUTICALS, PROBIOTICS, AND IV VITAMIN THERAPY... OH MY!

Let's take them one at a time:

#1 – NUTRACEUTICALS

OK, once you get past the self-consciously early-aughts pitch-meeting-era portmanteau (for anyone that *didn't* get the cool conflation, it's nutrition meets pharmaceuticals!), and, it's usually more of a pharmaceutically active nutrient than a nutritious pharmaceutical. As a more scientific definition, a nutraceutical has been described as "a product isolated from foods that is generally sold in medicinal forms not usually associated with food," and such product may be further defined as "a substance which has physiological benefit or provides protection against chronic diseases."[93] Another way to distinguish nutraceuticals from pharmaceuticals has been—at least historically—that nutraceuticals usually do not enjoy patent protection, whereas, of course, the pharmaceutical industry depends on patents[94]—so

---

93. Kalra EK. Nutraceutical – Definition and introduction. AAPS Pharm Sci. 2003;5:E25.
94. Zeisel SH. Regulation of "nutraceuticals" Science. 1999;285:1853–5.

that, at least for a good number of years, it can make enough money on a brand-name drug until the patent expires and then other companies can produce generic versions of the same compound. Pharmaceuticals also are regulated by the government, whereas nutraceuticals are not. But here is the key point:

Nutraceuticals Are Used for Purposes Other Than Essential Nutrition!

Huh? But, they're *nutra* – so, what are they used for? There are many answers, but the general tenor of them tend to revolve around prevention of chronic diseases, anti-aging uses, increasing life expectancy, and supporting the structure and/or function of certain parts of the body.

Here is something I started to touch on in our last chapter with supplements; and it really has to do with redefining what a supplement is. You see, generally, a nutraceutical is not a nutrient, because, according to the Oxford English Dictionary, that means "a substance that provides nourishment essential for the maintenance of life and for growth." And we already established they're neither a nutrient nor a pharmaceutical. If you're confused, don't be: Vitamins, minerals, and amino acids, for example, are supplements that are essential for your body. Nutraceuticals, while not essential for your body like the supplements mentioned above—and while not actually pharmaceuticals—may have real pharmaceutical value, modifying the natural course of diseases.

Arguably, after the rather amazing results showing that a "modified Mediterranean diet," supplemented with additional extra virgin oil and nuts, reduced deaths from heart attacks, olive oil could be termed a nutraceutical, but olive oil is so common that nobody would really consider it as such. However, if you read the fine print, the "extra olive oil" that was *added* to the study participants' diet was not just extra-virgin olive oil (EVOO) off the shelf. It was a special variety that was particularly rich in polyphenols. So, actually, it really was a nutraceutical, or a medical food, because it was either not commonly available, or it was specially grown, or otherwise modified, to enhance its pharmaceutical benefits.

WHAT IS A MEDICAL FOOD?

You may have heard about medical foods from friends or online. These are often placed in the same category as nutraceuticals. However, there are major differences. Medical foods were originally developed to help people with rare metabolic disorders. Now, of course, that market has vastly expanded. However, the FDA still has strict guidelines.[95, 96] It specifies that medical foods are foods which are specifically formulated for the dietary management of diseases or conditions with distinctive nutritional requirements that cannot be met solely by diet. Generally, a product has to meet the following criteria in order to be labeled a "medical food." It must be:

- A specific formulation (as opposed to a naturally-occurring foodstuff in its natural state) for oral or tube feeding;
- Labeled for the dietary management of a specific medical disorder, disease, or condition with distinctive nutritional requirements;
- Intended for use under medical supervision;
- Intended only for a patient receiving active and ongoing medical supervision for a condition requiring medical care on a recurring basis so that instructions on the use of the medical food can be provided.

Further, per the below-cited FDA regulations, the medical food must be used under medical supervision. Interestingly, unlike

---

95. US Food and Drug Administration. Compliance program guidance manual. Program 7321.002. Medical foods program -- import and domestic. Revised September 2008. Available at: http://www.fda.gov/downloads/Food/GuidanceComplianceRegulatoryInformation/ComplianceEnforcement/ucm073339.pdf
96. US Food and Drug Administration. Food. Guidance for industry: frequently asked questions about medical foods. Revised May 2007. Available at: http://www.fda.gov/Food/GuidanceComplianceRegulatoryInformation/GuidanceDocuments/MedicalFoods/ucm054048.htm.

dietary supplements, medical foods can be labeled for medical conditions such as Alzheimer disease. Here are three examples of medical foods which would never be allowed to be marketed as dietary supplements:

- Axona® (caprylic triglyceride): Marketed for dietary management of Alzheimer's disease. Caprylic triglyceride is a medium-chain triglyceride (MCT) found in coconut oil. As you may know, MCTs are all the rage among nutrition aficionados and bodybuilders.

- Limbrel® (flavocoxid): This drug is marketed for osteoarthritis. Because of its generic name, flavocoxid, which sounds remarkably similar to, like drugs, inhibitors such as celecoxib (Celebrex), it appears to be another COX-2 inhibitor (a powerful type of NSAID anti-inflammatory); however, instead, it is a proprietary blend of the flavonoid natural products baicalin and catechin (which comes from green tea).

- Foltx® (folic acid 2.5 mg, pyridoxine 25 mg, cyanocobalamin 2 mg): A mix of folate, Vitamin B6, and Vitamin B12, this preparation is marketed for hyperhomocysteinemia, which has been linked to cardiovascular disease. You wouldn't know it otherwise, but it's just three vitamins.

So, what are some nutraceuticals that I have been using to good effect in my practice?

Well, as you might have guessed, **Coenzyme Q10** has powerful benefits for the heart, as does **carnitine**. So does the amino acid **citrulline** (normally abundant in watermelons), which acts as a proxy for L-arginine, which helps to restore endothelial tone and function as a source of NO (nitric oxide). Nitric oxide, as you may recall, is one example of where free radicals are a good thing! As I told you in the last chapter, **curcumin** (from turmeric), **berberine**, and **cinnamon** are great at helping you control blood sugar. And whether you are diabetic or not, trust me, you need to control your blood sugar! Of course, you have already heard plenty about polyphenols, and the biggest among them is resveratrol. If you don't drink red wine, you may find it as a nutraceutical.

For more, you'll just have to come on into my office and ask me!

#2 – <u>PROBIOTICS</u>

There is currently a national obsession with probiotics. And, given the recognition that "our gut is our second brain," namely that the health of our gut microbiota very much seems to have great power over our overall health, the obsession seems understandable.

What Are Probiotics?

In a nutshell, probiotics are live cultures of organisms, usually bacteria, that are supposed to closely mirror the organisms in your body's normal flora (your body's natural gut microbiota). It is thought that these bacteria are health-promoting, and by supplying these in supplement form, you are replenishing the bacteria lost through natural processes, and especially through antibiotic treatment. Therefore, by taking probiotics, the theory goes, one can maintain a reasonable facsimile of a natural balance of the gut microbiota that normally exists. Some of these probiotics are readily familiar to you, such as the *Acidophilus* species, *Lactobacillus*, and *Bifidobacterium* species. The reason these sound so familiar to you is that they are in dairy products, particularly yogurt, cultured milks such as kefir and buttermilk, and, of course, the majority of the probiotic capsules you buy.

However, the probiotic organisms are not limited solely to bacteria: they also include yeasts! The yeast *Saccharomyces boulardii* is a very close cousin to *Saccharomyces cerevisiae*, the yeast we know and love that makes dough rise. However, the species difference supposedly gives it some beneficial properties as a probiotic, such as utility in treating antibiotic-associated diarrhea.

While antibiotics are overprescribed in *general*, they are necessary in many cases. Yet some of them unfortunately have nasty gastrointestinal side effects because they annihilate the native GI flora. So, by administering the right kind of probiotics to ease the side effects that the antibiotics often cause, this gives the integrative medicine practitioner like myself a decided advantage over the conventional doctor.

What Are Prebiotics?

Often confused with *pro*biotics, *pre*biotics are substances that you can consume which are *not bacteria*, but which select for, and favor, the growth of good bacteria (like your normal flora) as opposed to bad bacteria, e.g., pathogens, or disease-causing bacteria. A good example of a prebiotic is thought to be the sugar alcohol, erythritol, which is nearly as sweet as sugar, without the deleterious effects.

#3 – <u>IV VITAMIN THERAPY</u>

IV Vitamin Therapy is something that I have been doing for a few years, but as sort of a miniature laboratory to test out different special formulations. Sure, I offer the Myers' Cocktail, which is a blend of B vitamins, which today has become best known for reviving people after hangovers. Sure, it brings in the customers, and I have certainly gotten my share of publicity for my celebrity clients being able to party like the rock stars they are and then do it all over again. However, that is not the overarching intent of my work.

What I have been working on, with the help of my select brain trust of formulation chemists, scientific advisers, and the patients who have tested out our early formulations through my program, is, first of all, an optimized methodology for doing chelation therapy to reduce side effects, risks, and improve overall results; and second, a specifically-compounded IV infusion that combines the best of chelation therapy with the latest proprietary anti-aging, heart-healthy treatment methodologies.

SECTION 3

PIONEER

CHAPTER 15

PIONEER

The first part of the journey you took with me in this book involved my telling you how you could accurately assess your odds of getting a heart attack (in essence, to PREDICT).

The second leg of the adventure gave you what I think is a lot of good reasons to start enjoying life again by learning some of what I have been teaching you to PREVENT heart attacks. These represent some very preliminary, but encouraging insights, into boosting your chances of living to be a hundred years old without a heart attack.

And third, right here, is to PIONEER new methods of combating heart attacks. Sure, everybody says words like "pioneer" all the time. Especially people who start web startups! 'Cause it's a cool word, like "innovate," "spearhead," and "bootstrap." Some people also know it as a recognizable brand of car stereo, and those in Southern California might recall it being associated with fried chicken outlets. But I post the dictionary definition for the word **"pioneer"** on the following pages for a very good reason:

pioneer[1]

/ˌpīəˈnir/

noun
1. a person who is among the first to explore or settle a new country or area.
   synonyms: settler, colonist, colonizer, frontiersman/frontierswoman, explorer, trailblazer, discoverer
   'the pioneers of the Wild West'
2. a person who is among the first to research and develop a new area of knowledge or activity.
   'a famous pioneer of a vaccine'

verb
1. develop or be the first to use or apply (a new method, area of knowledge, or activity).
   synonyms: develop, introduce, evolve, start, begin, launch, instigate, initiate, lay the ground work for,
   institute, establish, to take the initiative, create, establish

Origin of pioneer
French *pionnier* from Old French *peonier*, foot soldier from *peon*
1. being one of the first of its kind
2. of or characteristic of the settlers of a new territory

pi·o·neer
/ˌpīəˈnir/
noun
1. One who ventures into unknown or unclaimed territory to settle.
2. One who opens up new areas of thought, research, or development: *a pioneer in aviation.*
3. A soldier who performs construction and demolition work in the field to facilitate troop
   movements.
4. A species that is typically among the first to become established in a bare, open, or disturbed area.
adjective
1. Of, relating to, or characteristic of early settlers: *the pioneer spirit.*
2. Leading the way; trailblazing: *a pioneer treatment for cancer.*
verb

pi·o·neered, pi·o·neer·ing, pi·o·neers
verb

transitive
1. **a.** To venture into (an area) or prepare (a way): *rockets that pioneered outer space.*
   b. To settle (a region).
2. To initiate or participate in the development of: *surgeons who pioneered organ transplants.*
verb

intransitive
To act as a pioneer: *pioneered in development of the laser.*

Origin of pioneer
French *pionnier from* Old French *peonier foot soldier from peon from* Medieval
Latin *pedō pedōn- from* Late Latin *one who has broad feet from* Latin *pēs ped- foot.*
[1]pioneer. (n.d.). Retrieved February 20th, 2019, from https://www.yourdictionary.com/PIONEER

Because, while "pioneering" is very appealing, and seemingly, quite rewarding, look at the etymology of the word: It goes back to the Latin for "foot," as in "foot soldiers," who established their presence in a new town by marching into it. The word "pawn," as in the chess piece, as you see from the graphic, is directly related. While not glamorous the way the king or queen is, the pawns are integral to chess strategy. Here, the pawns, the "foot soldiers," are scientific researchers in laboratories all over the world who have the ability to connect and collaborate not only with one another, but with those of use in clinical practice in doctors' offices and hospitals, and in ways that they, and I, would have never have previously imagined. The ability to "translate research into results," as I call it, has happened at a faster pace than I can ever recall. What does that mean? That means a researcher at a teaching university, such as UCLA, can design a new experimental drug, put it into clinical trials, and get results out of those trials in a few years, as opposed to ten or 15, especially if the drugs are so-called "biologics," such as monoclonal antibodies, as so many of our new medications are. Sometimes, that few years can be expedited for "compassionate use" trials (patients who are in severe health crises, and whose conditions are thought to be terminal without these experimental treatments).

BUT WHAT'S NEW ON THE HORIZON?

1. NEW DIAGNOSTIC BIOMARKERS

The discovery of some novel diagnostic markers over the past two years is one of the most exciting diagnostic breakthroughs in years. These biomarkers (which constitute an important part of my algorithm) allow for a much better assessment (what in the medical community is referred to as "risk stratification") of existing or future cardiovascular disease.

One example of these exciting biomarkers is ST-2. ST-2 is a surrogate biomarker for many types of heart disease: It binds directly to the well-known IL-33 ("IL" indicates "interleukin") ligand. It has been proven to be far superior even to some of the standard biomarkers that hospitals use to test to see if you have had a heart attack, such as troponins, at least for the heart attack type called the "non-STEMI."

When it comes to stratifying patients in the hospital for risk of heart attack, the biomarker CRP (C-Reactive Protein) is often used, as it is a surrogate marker of global inflammation. Galectin-3 is also typically helpful in triaging high-risk patients. But, guess what? ST-2 completely makes both CRP and Galectin-3, in the context of risk stratification, look practically useless! Further, while studies to characterize ST-2 were being done, and its amazing utility began to become understood, the investigators came to realize that perhaps ST-2's greatest predictive value lay not in predicting a "heart attack," or "myocardial infarction," as we docs usually call it," but in identifying a very insidious, and, unfortunately, quite common issue: congestive heart failure (CHF).

You see, ST-2 not only identifies patients who have CHF and might not have known it, but, by measuring precise *changes in their ST-2 levels*, we might be able to help them head off more serious problems which often occur in the setting of CHF. What do I mean by that?

Well, as a threshold issue, CHF is an inflammatory disease. It also has a pulmonary component, so we have to make sure our patients' lungs don't get congested and get fluid backup. Also, people with CHF are much more likely to have an MI—oops, I mean, a heart attack—because of the inflammation in the myocytes, as well as the blood vessels, that has been a pre-existing condition. So by checking ST-2 (and other inflammatory biomarkers), we can try to head off a disaster. I would also try to prescribe anti-inflammatories, including supplements.

And, by the way, if you've already had a heart attack, usually within the first 24 to 48 hours after the heart attack has occurred, there will inevitably be some remodeling of the ventricular walls that takes place. As a very nice review article puts it: "Cardiac remodeling can be described as a physiologic and pathologic response that may follow myocardial infarction (MI), pressure overload (aortic stenosis, hypertension), inflammatory heart muscle disease (myocarditis), idiopathic dilated cardiomyopathy or volume overload conditions (valvular regurgitation). It refers to alteration of ventricular architecture."

Remodeling of your heart is not an easy process: It takes two phases. The early phase is the first 72 hours, and the "late phase" refers to the next 72 hours. (The same review article states these figures.) At this point, in case anyone is wondering, this kind of "remodeling" is not like some easy project your heart goes out and does on the weekend at "Heart Depot." I don't know where they got the "72-hour" figure, but with contractors *I've* seen these days, lemme tell ya, everything *always* takes *twice* as long as they say. You just have to build that in. Martha Stewart would not be saying, "It's a good thing!"

But seriously, folks, ST-2 is just one of the many exciting new diagnostic innovations I have implemented in my practice. Because CHF is such a huge issue, we have been looking at other tests that help us in research for our HF patients. One very interesting area of research being currently in the works is how patients with HF utilize energy differently than patients without HF: As the heart fails, it is less and less able to use its chief fuel source—oxidation of fatty acids, and instead, it shifts to using ketone bodies. This complete shift in fuel use is reminiscent of how cancer cells differentially rely on glycolysis vs. non-cancer cells (the famed Warburg effect). By exploiting these sorts of vulnerabilities, we can look to design drugs. The field of drug design is now one where drugs may literally be designed around enzyme-active sites, or receptors. Drugs may thus be designed to fit like a glove.

2. PROMISING NEW THERAPEUTIC APPROACHES

Stem-Cell Therapies for The Heart

You may have heard about it in the context of heart failure patients receiving them. But, stem cell therapies have also been used to beneficial effect on patients who have suffered heart attacks. Why is this? Because after an MI, the muscle cells have been damaged or destroyed, and those heart muscle cells, unfortunately, just do not grow back by themselves. But the stem cells, as you probably know, are *pluripotent*, which means they have that wonderful, magic ability to grow other heart muscle cells! That is why the process has shown some promise with post-MI patients.

The Promise of Genetic Engineering and Gene Therapy to Stop Heart Attacks

We keep being told as a society that genetic engineering, or gene therapy, will be able to cure all the horrible diseases that ail us; and heart disease certainly qualifies. When the human genome was sequenced in 2003, it was thought that scientists would be able to easily genetically engineer solutions to the major inherited diseases first (diseases where we knew what genes were affected, such as sickle-cell anemia, cystic fibrosis, or Tay-Sachs disease), and then proceed to the more multi-factorial diseases (ones which are partly genetically determined, and partly impacted by environmental factors, such as heart disease and cancer). So, what's taking everyone so long? What's the issue, guys? Other than this being a silly and facetious statement, there have actually been some very promising developments in gene therapy lately – such as a recent study out of UCLA that identified a gene that could be used to essentially help pump plaque out of blocked arteries. Another ongoing interesting research is engineering genes involved in oxidation and modification of LDL molecules, as well as modification of the endothelium and the glycocalyx (see Section I).

3. MACHINE LEARNING

This is not just the broadly-thrown-around term "artificial intelligence," but it is better described as "neural networks," or "expert systems." These systems, the best-known of which are exemplified by IBM's "Watson" computer, are able to "learn" by aggregating insanely large numbers of data points, and are then fed "diagnostic" medical information. However, the amount of data that Watson has been fed in addition to these data points includes exceedingly large databases of other patient diagnostic data. Perhaps it also includes unsolved cases. But the "deep learning" diagnostic abilities of such neural networks have become so good that, to some doctors, they are almost frightening.

Imagine, if you will, a computer that is able to use hundreds of thousands of MRIs and other imaging studies, as well as lab results for a wide variety of different tests, in a series of many hundreds of thousands of breast cancer patients. Then imagine a hospital treatment team receiving a patient with advanced breast cancer. The team obtains an MRI, bone scan, and a whole battery of tests. The oncologist recommends a course of chemotherapy, but the computer, receiving the same data, predicts the patient will die in 11 days, and recommends hospice and palliative care. The patient dies in 12 days. Stories such as this are now no longer fictional. And with the stakes very high for insurers in such high-value areas as cardiology, I have no doubt that this is happening in our field as well.

What is scary is the computer (usually) cannot provide a reason for the prediction. It just takes everything together and spits out a result. Utilization review departments of insurance companies (the bean counters who come into the hospitals, stick their noses into the doctors' charts and question the doctors' independent medical judgments) absolutely love these new "deep learning" computers, because they have the potential to improve the insurers' bottom line. But the prospect of a computer overruling a doctor's judgment without even being able to give anyone a reason for its decision is scaring a lot of people, especially my fellow doctors.

But, as I understand it, Amazon is working on an expert system that will do the same thing—and provide reasoning for the decision behind it. One wonders if it will also use the synthesized voice when delivering the "reasoned opinion." I can just see it now: "Dr. Alexa predicts that, based on declining serum albumin levels, the patient is expected to expire within 5.3 days. Would you like me to send an electronic prescription to the patient's pharmacy or print the patient's chart for you?"

CHAPTER 16

PUTTING IT ALL TOGETHER

A LOOK INTO THE FUTURE

People have asked me what I think the future of cardiology might look like. And, as I hope you might imagine, I am optimistic.

The practice of medicine has been going through a complete change over the past 3-5 years and will continue to do so in the next 20 years, thanks mostly to the technology. Gone will be doctor's waiting rooms and even though clinics will still exist, there would be only a handful of them (and mostly as part of the hospitals). The diagnosis and treatment will move online.

Using HIPPA-compliant websites, and remote, handless technologies such as blue-tooth, the doctors will see and "visit" their patients online, listen to their patient's heart using a Wi-FI enabled stethoscope and see the patient's 12-lead ECG that has been transmitted to the doctor via an extremely small patch on the patient's body or even implanted under the skin of the patient. Even critically sick patients in intensive care units of the hospitals will be managed remotely via the help of "Robot Doctors." Sounds like Sci-Fi? Well, it is not. The above technologies have already been created and tested and it is a matter of time before it becomes implemented globally.

In about 5 to 7 years, you will be able to monitor your entire body (how your kidneys, heart and liver are functioning as well as your hormone levels in addition to your heart rate, blood pressure, temperature, respiratory rate and level of hydration which are already available. Furthermore, your watch (or a patch implanted in you) will instantly notify the emergency personnel should it detect you are about to have a heart attack or stroke. Imagine a scenario where your doctor calls you to immediately take an aspirin while an ambulance arrives at your doorstep to transport you to the closest hospital MINUTES before you are about to have a heart attack or a stroke! This is not a fantasy anymore.

In regards to the future of prevention, in the short term there will be a polypill with everything you need to prevent a heart attack if you are at risk. Sound naïve? Well, it is not. My center, in collaboration with others, is conducting research as I am writing this. In the long term, however, my hope is that no one would ever again need to use medication, as genetic engineering and stem cell therapies will correct and treat all form of cardiac abnormalities before they cause disease.

THE B-100 METHOD

Over the past 9 years, my team and I have been working on a project called ***The B-100 Method***. The name is derived from our goal of having people live to **Be 100** without ever having had a heart attack.

The B-100 Method, if I had to reduce it to simplest terms, involves a painstakingly chosen, comprehensive battery of tests and data points/inputs (currently numbering over 100), which enables us to predict, I believe, with greater specificity than any other model, a patient's <u>risk</u> of sustaining a heart attack or cardiovascular event—and then, if the patient has a positive result, of predicting roughly when that CV event will occur, based on certain values within the model.

The B-100-Method is, at the present time, a series of diagnostic tests, or data points. However, the ultimate objective of the Method is the much-bandied-about, but rarely properly understood term, "personalized medicine." That is, to utilize, to our full ability, as our patients' doctors, the full battery of tests, and the information such tests have afforded us with respect to each patient's own genetic susceptibilities and frailties—and then to combine that information with the research information we have currently at our disposal to enable us not only to use the pharmacopoeia we have right now, but to develop exciting, innovative solutions for our patients. Custom-formulated solutions, if you will, which are informed by the individual results of that patient's B-100 Method.

My goal is that no matter where the field of cardiology takes us in the future, the B-100 method would become an integral part of it and as the technology and new discoveries are made, the B-100 community will grow with it as it will continue to further refine and develop the Method that I have created for the benefit of all concerned. And, with that said, I will dedicate my life to showing the world that we can all live to B-100 without having a heart attack!

Look out for more exciting information on B-100 in the very near future.

APPENDIX A

CHOLESTEROL

A sterol is a steroid which is an alcohol. Since these are large molecules, sterols are solid alcohols, despite the "alcohol" connotation as a liquid. **I understand that not all of you may understand chemistry: I just want you to look at the structural similarities and differences.** Remember, every vertex is a C (Carbon) atom. Every carbon atom has four bonds it can make, either to an H (Hydrogen) atom, which is implied where not explicitly shown), or another vertex (Carbon), or another kind of atom, e.g., O (oxygen), which will be shown in the figures below. All figures are public domain:

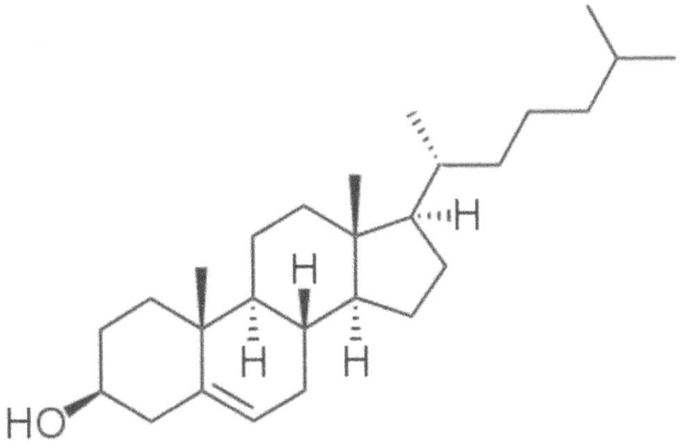

Fig.1 Cholesterol Structure

Cholesterol structure. The "-ol," is the "-OH" group on the left side.

Cholesterol is also the precursor of bile acids, such as cholic acid, below, which are necessary for the proper digestion and emulsification of lipids in your small intestine. Within the liver, in the hepatocytes (liver cells), some of that cholesterol gets converted into bile acids like the **cholic acid** shown below.

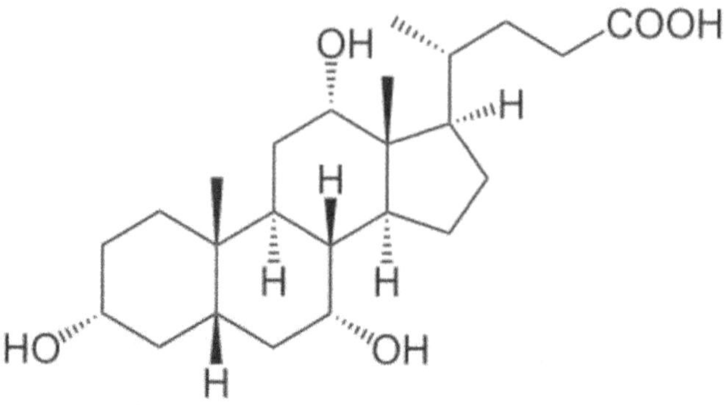

Fig.2 Cholic Acid Structure

Cholic acid (a bile acid) **structure**, above. See how similar it looks to cholesterol? What are the differences? For one thing, the alcohol, "-OH" group is sticking out of the plane in the cholesterol, but *into* the plane of the paper in cholic acid. That means the atoms are facing downward relative to the ring. That actually is a thing. It makes a difference. That's why we draw them that way. For another thing, on cholic acid, see the big H sticking up out of the plane at you where ring A joins ring B? [The first two rings (lower rings) left to right are called "A" and "B"; the second two (upper rings), "C" and "D".]

Notice how that H is *not* there in the structure of cholesterol? What *is* there, directly adjacent to where the H would have gone? Well, for those of you who don't know, you see the little line inside Ring B right where it joins Ring A? Remember that every vertex is a carbon atom, and every carbon atom can have four bonds. That extra line is called a [C=C] **double bond**. Double bonds can also join carbon atoms to oxygen and nitrogen atoms too. Carbon can even form triple bonds with other carbons, although those are strictly linear, not bent. Why are double bonds important biologically? Because double bonds are more commonly called **unsaturations**, as in—you guessed it: unsaturated fats.

Pro tip: When a hydrocarbon chain has no double bonds, it is called "fully saturated."

Monounsaturated fats = fats with only one "unsaturation," or one double bond.

Polyunsaturated fats have multiple double bonds.

The *arrangement* of the atoms in space *on the double bond* also affects its physical and chemical properties:

cis-2-butene	*trans*-2-butene
The H's (or the CH3's, for that matter), are on the same side, or *cis*, to each other	The H's (or the CH3's, for that matter), are on the *opposite* side or *trans*, of one another.

Now, extend this principle to its natural state, because we don't eat butene. We eat butyric acid though—pretty close.

We eat **saturated fatty acids**, like butyric acid (butter) and stearic acid (steer, beef). And we eat **unsaturated fatty acids** when we cook with natural vegetable oils. These contain mixtures of different monounsaturated and polyunsaturated fatty acids, which have their double bonds in the normal *cis* configuration, meaning the carbon atoms are on the same sides as each other. These double bonds are more easily subject to auto-oxidation—

which is not good, just as oxidized LDL is not good—explaining why sometimes natural oils go rancid quickly, while partially hydrogenated oils do not.

When you **partially hydrogenate** oils by adding hydrogen across those double bonds, you change them to single bonds (making them "saturated,") and changing the melting point of the oil, and the more solid a fat you get. This is how margarine is made. So, a completely hydrogenated fat is solid at room temperature. But most of the time on labels, you will see "partially hydrogenated soybean oil," which means the mixture is lower in *trans* fatty acids. Fast-food companies and big packaged food manufacturer like *trans* fats because they have a longer shelf life. Unfortunately, when you consume them, you have a shorter **"self" life.** This is because *trans* fats raise your LDL-C and lower your HDL-C.

APPENDIX B

MECHANISMS BY WHICH ACUTE STRESS CAUSES HEART ATTACKS

What are the *mechanisms* responsible? It may seem obvious to the casual observer that these are seriously stressful events, and, as such, too much stress placed on the heart would naturally cause the heart to "give out." However, in today's world of evidence-based medicine, and in cases where, for example, there is a need to prove more conclusively *how* the sequence of events played out that ended in a patient's untimely demise, a deeper understanding of their inner workings, and, perhaps most importantly to the readers of this book, if the stressful events have already occurred, and stopping them is impossible, how to intercede in the biochemical pathways that we think are responsible for leading from said stressful events to a future heart attack. This is the sort of analysis I have been doing that is typical of my B-100 program. Obviously, every cardiologist—indeed, every doctor—will tell you it is important to reduce your stress. I will, too. But I also aim to get at exactly the reasons "why" and "how" stress causes heart attacks, and then show you the latest in what we know about how to protect yourself against having a stress-related heart attack.

How does mental stress cause *physical* cardiovascular issues?

Picture for a few minutes this little suburban scenario. Let's go back to the basics of what might happen in the course of your "feeling stressed" without having a major catastrophe like an earthquake in the picture. Let's imagine, for example, that you're Bob, a Creative Director at an ad agency, and you were preparing for a big presentation for a client in the morning, so you pulled an all-nighter because you just knew you could knock their socks off with your new design concept—and this would get you a raise or a promotion, which you were hoping to use to buy your wife something special for her birthday. You knew she was looking forward to a nice surprise at dinner tonight, because you'd dropped hints about it, and you always went above and beyond what everyone expected of you. Your storyboards are brilliant, but you doze off for a split second on the freeway while driving to work, which is all it takes for you to rear-end another vehicle (automatically your fault, now your insurance rates are going up), which—although you are not traveling at high speed, jolts you awake with a sickening, shocking feeling that has you gasping for breath, clutching your chest, and in a sheer panic.

But wait, there's more. You see the ominous black and white outline of a Highway Patrol cruiser swooping in, the finality of its whoop-whoop sealing your fate. You feel like you are about to pass out, but your cell phone rings, and, of course, it's your boss: "Dammit, Bob! You told me you had this amazing presentation, and I'm sitting here with the client. What the heck..." You, meanwhile, can hardly eke out more than a few distressed words: "But Mr. Quackenbush! You don't understand what just happened to me!" Your boss responds: "Bob, just because you've suddenly gotten all on this whole *fitness* kick with that cardiologist, what's his name, Dr. Brilliantini?" ["No, Dr. Bereliani, he's helping me B-100," you struggle to correct him.] "B-100? Is that a vitamin? Well, from the way you sound, he's obviously having you do high-impact cardio to start your workday—very inconvenient with our business hours, by the way—and listen to yourself, you can hardly breathe! So, you keep on doing that, and you tell the good doctor Barely Any you already have the "Barely Any" plan right here: Barely Any *job*, that is, because if you keep on doing his crazy aerobics plan like you did this morning instead of making a presentation for a top-tier client, so help me, Bob." Once again, Bob's heart was pounding at what felt like a mile a minute, and then it started to skip beats. He felt nauseated. "Mr. Quackenbush, it was all an accident, literally. I was *in* an accident. If I could *explain...*"

THE SYMPATHETIC NERVOUS SYSTEM

Obviously, the three catecholamine neurotransmitters are extremely powerful compounds, and are pivotal in many functions of the human body. But two of them, **epinephrine** and **norepinephrine**, are especially known for the body's so-called *fight-or-flight* response, which is controlled by the *sympathetic nervous system*. This part of the nervous system raises heart rate and blood pressure in response to **adrenaline (= epinephrine, the terms are interchangeable)**. The third catecholamine, *dopamine*, is a powerful brain neurotransmitter, functioning as the basis for your brain's reward system. All three of them are synthesized by your adrenal glands (although they can be made by other parts of your body as well). The sympathetic nervous system produces greater amounts of epinephrine in response to fear to mobilize your body to be able to run faster (away from a lion in the old days, for example), so that epinephrine dilates your bronchioles, enabling freer breathing —this is why epinephrine is very helpful during an asthma attack—has a positive inotropic effect on your heart (increased contractile force on the heart muscle), increases your blood pressure, and increases your heart rate.

ACUTE STRESS AND SUDDEN CARDIAC DEATH

It is perhaps a truism that some people who experience severe, acute episodes of stress, such as survivors of major life events, e.g., earthquakes, hurricanes, tornadoes, or victims of violent crime and trauma, suffer massive heart attacks which result in sudden cardiac death (SCD). "Their heart just couldn't take it." The degree to which this characterization has approached the status of folklore has not been lost on George Engel, the author of

"Sudden and Rapid Death During Psychological Stress: Folklore or Folk Wisdom?" a seminal paper on the subject exploring the categorization of psychosocial stressors involved in SCD,[97] which purports to neatly divide said psychosocial stressors into eight (8) discrete categories, depending on when the SCD occurred:

(1) On the impact of the collapse or death of a close person
(2) During acute grief
(3) On threat of loss of a close person
(4) During mourning or on an anniversary
(5) On the loss of status or self-esteem
(6) Personal danger or threat of injury
(7) After the danger is over
(8) Reunion, triumph, or happy ending

According to Engel, what is *common* to all of these items is that "they involve events impossible for the victims to ignore and to which their response is overwhelming excitation or giving up, or both." He proposes that "this combination provokes neurovegetative responses, involving both the flight-fight and conservation-withdrawal systems, which are conducive to lethal cardiac events, particularly in individuals with preexisting cardiovascular disease; other modes of death, however, were also noted."

BEREAVEMENT

With respect to items (1) and (2), extending that one step further, another very common source of acute stress is bereavement: the loss of a loved one, especially when sudden and unexpected, has tended to cause higher rates of SCD in the surviving spouse. In a large prospective study of 95,647 widowed persons, the highest relative mortality occurred immediately after bereavement, with a more than two-fold higher risk for men and three-fold higher risk for women. After the first month, mortality rates returned

---

97. Engel, G. Sudden and Rapid Death During Psychological Stress: Folklore or Folk Wisdom? Ann Intern Med. 1971;74(5):771-783.

to normal population levels.[98] One could certainly argue that sympathetic overload might be in play in causing these deaths, but what about coronary artery disease? How do the two interact? Look at the diagram below. It's quite an interesting explanation. **And what about patients who *had* no history of CVD before, but simply witnessed their loved one die, then suffered a massive heart attack? They literally just died of a broken heart!**

Glad you asked. That's what we call Takotsubo cardiomyopathy. It's actually not *usually* fatal. But it happens in response to "a broken heart." It is much more common in older female patients who have just lost their husbands, and results from sympathetic nervous system overstimulation. If you look at these patients, they generally do *not* have atherosclerosis.

<u>Mechanism for Sympathetic Nervous System Overstimulation Causing SCD:</u>

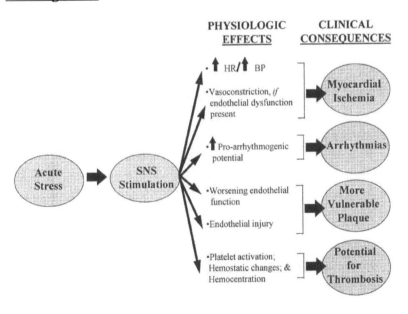

---

98. Kaprio J, Koskenvuo M, Rita H. Mortality after bereavement: a prospective study of 95,647 widowed persons. Am J Public Health. 1987 Mar;77(3):283-7.

The diagram on the previous page shows a "Schematic of pathophysiological effects of acute psychosocial stress. Sympathetic nervous system (SNS) stimulation emanating from acute stress leads to a variety of effects, ranging from heart rate and blood pressure stimulation to direct effects on coronary vascular endothelium. Clinical consequences of these effects include development of myocardial ischemia, cardiac arrhythmias, and fostering of more vulnerable coronary plaques and hemostatic changes. These changes form a substrate for development of acute myocardial infarction and sudden cardiac death."[99]

DON'T LOOK BACK IN ANGER

It may seem simple, but don't get angry—or try not to get as angry. Because people who got the angriest paid the ultimate price, according to a major study.[100]

Out of over 1,600 patients, those on a 7-point scale (1=calm, 7=enraged) was used, with anger episodes defined as scores ≥5. After an episode of anger, the relative risk of myocardial infarction was increased >2-fold.

99. Rozanski, A, Blumenthal, JA, Kaplan J. Impact of Psychological Factors on the Pathogenesis of Cardiovascular Disease and Implications for Therapy. Circulation. 1999;99:2192-2217
100. Mittleman MA, Maclure M, Sherwood JB, Mulry RP, Tofler GH, Jacobs SC, Friedman R, Benson H, Muller JE, for the Determinants Of Myocardial Infarction Onset Study Investigators. Triggering of acute myocardial infarction onset by episodes of anger. Circulation. 1995;92:1720–1725.

PHYSIOLOGIC
EFFECTS

CLINICAL
CONSEQUENCES

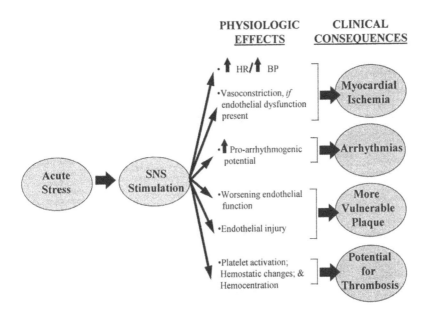

HYPERSENSITIVITY TO SYMPATHETIC STIMULATION

Do people tell you that you're just too sensitive for your own good? Maybe they're right! Maybe you are just hypersensitive to the stimulation of epinephrine and norepinephrine of your own sympathetic nervous system. And as a result, you're called a "hot reactor" instead of a "cold reactor".[101] Unfortunately, this is not a good thing, and renders you more likely to suffer SCD through the mechanisms described above. So what can you do?

101. Keys A, Longstreet T, Blackburn H, Brozek J, Anderson JT, Simonson E. Mortality and coronary heart disease among men studied for 23 years. Arch Intern Med. 1971;128:201–214.

INDEX

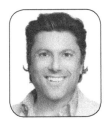

About Dr. B

Dr. Arash Bereliani, also known as "Dr. B The Heart Doc", is a world-renowned expert leading the field in Preventative and Functional Cardiovascular Disease. He is a Board Certified Cardiologist and Associate Clinical Professor of Medicine and Cardiology at UCLA School of Medicine. Dr. Bereliani is the current Medical Director of The Beverly Hills Institute of Cardiology and Preventive Medicine where he has successfully treated some of the most complex and life-threatening cardiac conditions for over 15 years.

Dr. Bereliani's practice is uniquely positioned amongst an extremely small group of cardiologists worldwide, who possess in-depth knowledge of functional and orthomolecular medicine, to apply an integrative approach that seeks to use all scientific and proven methods available (not just medication) to treat heart disease.

As a leader in the field of Preventive Cardiology, he specializes in incorporating the latest cutting-edge research, advanced genetic testing along with highly specialized and sophisticated biomarkers to assess an individual's chance of developing significant cardiovascular disease within specified subsequent years. Dr. B then creates a personalized, comprehensive treatment approach for each individual patient. In treating patients, both those with and without cardiovascular disease, he combines the best of traditional and integrative medicine.

Dr. B is actively researching the latest and most advanced cardiac monitoring technologies, many of which are being used in his practice. In addition to working in private practice for over 15 years, Dr. B has served as a Clinical Associate Professor of Medicine and Cardiology at UCLA's Geffen School of Medicine since 2003. He is also on the staff and part of Cedars-Sinai Medical Center's renowned Center of Excellence.

Dr. B received his medical degree from Finch University of Health Sciences in Chicago, where he was ranked number one in his graduating class (of 192 students), receiving numerous awards and honors that included being inducted into the Alpha Omega Alpha (AOA) Medical Honor Society, a fraternity to which only the top 10% of medical students in the country are invited. He went on to complete his internal medicine and cardiology training at Ronald Reagan UCLA Medical Center.

Dr. B strives to give back to his community through his fundraising efforts to further heart disease, cancer and Alzheimer's research. Equally important, he created a non-profit organization to help patients with no or low income get access to heart disease testing.

In his free time he enjoys spending time with his beautiful wife, daughter and their two dogs, and loves to raise his adrenaline by getting behind the wheel at the race track!